www.harcourt-international.com

Bringing you products from all Harcourt Health Sciences companies including Baillière Tindall, Churchill Livingstone, Mosby and W.B. Saunders

- ❍ **Browse** for latest information on new books, journals and electronic products

- ❍ **Search** for information on over 20 000 published titles with full product information including tables of contents and sample chapters

- ❍ **Keep up to date** with our extensive publishing programme in your field by registering with **eAlert** or requesting postal updates

- ❍ **Secure online ordering** with prompt delivery, as well as full contact details to order by phone, fax or post

- ❍ **News** of special feature

D1157656

If you are based in the follow...... countries, please..... : the country-specific site to receive full details of product availability and local ordering information

USA: www.harcourthealth.com

Canada: www.harcourtcanada.com

Australia: www.harcourt.com.au

 Baillière Tindall 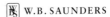 CHURCHILL LIVINGSTONE ▶️ Mosby 🅆🅂 W.B. SAUNDERS

Managing Communication in Health Care

For Baillière Tindall

Senior Commissioning Editor: Jacqueline Curthoys
Project Development Manager: Karen Gilmour
Project Manager: Jane Dingwall
Design Direction: George Ajayi/Judith Wright

Managing Communication in Health Care

Edited by

Mark Darley RGN BA(Hons) MA

Operational Services Manager, Faculty of Health – Essex Campus, South Bank University, Harold Wood, Ramford, UK

Foreword by

Christina Edwards MBA RGN RHV

Regional Director of Nursing and Workforce Development, NHS Northern and Yorkshire Regional Office, Durham, UK

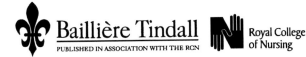

EDINBURGH LONDON NEW YORK PHILADELPHIA ST LOUIS SYDNEY TORONTO 2002

Baillière Tindall
An imprint of Harcourt Publishers Limited

© Harcourt Publishers Limited 2002

❧ is a registered trademark of Harcourt Publishers Limited

The right of Mark Darley to be identified as the editor of this work has been asserted by him in accordance with the Copyright, Designs and Patents Act 1988

First published 2002

ISBN 0 7020 2413 9

British Library Cataloguing in Publication Data
A catalogue record for this book is available from the British Library

Library of Congress Cataloging in Publication Data
A catalog record for this book is available from the Library of Congress

Note
Medical knowledge is constantly changing. As new information becomes available, changes in treatment, procedures, equipment and the use of drugs become necessary. The editor and contributors and the publishers have taken care to ensure that the information given in this text is accurate and up to date. However, readers are strongly advised to confirm that the information, especially with regard to drug usage, complies with the latest legislation and standards of practice.

The
publisher's
policy is to use
**paper manufactured
from sustainable forests**

Printed in China by RDC Group Limited

Six Steps to Effective Management series

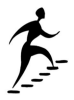

Managing the Business of Health Care
Edited by Julie Hyde and Frances Cooper

Managing and Implementing Decisions in Health Care
Edited by Ann Young and Mary Cooke

Managing and Leading Innovation in Health Care
Edited by Elizabeth Howkins and Cynthia Thornton

Managing Communication in Health Care
Edited by Mark Darley

Managing Diversity and Inequality in Health Care
Edited by Carol Baxter

Managing and Supporting People in Health Care
Edited by Margaret Buttigieg and Surrinder Kaur

Series editor: Ann Young

About the series

The Six Steps to Effective Management series comes at a time when the speed and extent of change within health care have rarely been greater, and the challenges facing nurses and everyone working within the health care sector are extensive. The series identifies and discusses those challenges and suggests ways of managing them. It aims to be unique in that it links theory with practice through the application of evidence where available and includes case studies which build on sound and relevant theoretical material.

All nurses are required by the clinical governance agenda to have a grasp of management principles. The *Six Steps to Effective Management* series is both practical enough to appeal to the practitioner and theoretical enough to be useful to those undertaking courses at undergraduate or diploma level. The books are relevant to all nurses.

The series comprises six volumes that are carefully constructed to contain a mix of theoretical and practical approaches, research and case studies, including a variety of perspectives from different sectors of health care. Each volume is relevant, realistic and practical to encourage reflection and critical thinking to prepare readers for flexible and adaptable styles of management.

For more information on this series please contact: Harcourt Health Sciences Health Professions Marketing Department on +44 20 7424 4200.

Contents

Six Steps to **Effective Management**

Contents

Contributors

Helen Brett MSc RGN DipN(Lon) CertEd
Senior Lecturer, Faculty of Nursing, Midwifery and Social Work,
Canterbury Christ Church University College, Kent

Mark Darley RGN BA(Hons) MA
Operational Services Manager, Faculty of Health – Essex
Campus, South Bank University, Harold Wood, Romford

Linda Ewles MA MSc BSc
Freelance Public Health Specialist in Communication, Hallatrow, Bristol

Yvonne Hill BA MA RGN RNT
Principal Lecturer in Nursing Studies, Faculty of Nursing,
Midwifery and Social Work, Canterbury Christ Church University
College, Kent

Catriona King MB BCh BaO MBA
Strategic Advisor in Primary Care to Dean of Faculty of Health,
South Bank University and Honorary Senior Tutor in Primary Care at
St George's Medical School, London

Janet Knowles BSc MEd MSc CPsychol
Director, Qualis Ltd, London

Cath Lovatt BSc(Hons) DipM MCIM Chartered Marketer
Healthcare Public Relations Consultant, Atlas Public Relations Ltd, Leeds

Brenda Maslen RMN DipN CertEd MEd RNT
Freelance Lecturer, Bessacarr Grange, Doncaster

Fiona McGreur

Anne Palmer MA BEd(Hons) RN RM RNT
Chair, Department of Community and Collaborative Practice,
School of Integrated Health, University of Westminster, London

Stuart Skyte DMS
Head of Communications, UKCC, London

Mike Tatlow MSc PG Cert FEATC DCR CertCT SRR
Senior Lecturer in Diagnostic Radiography, Division of Professions Allied
to Medicine, Faculty of Health, Southbank University, London

Colleen Wedderburn Tate MSc BA DMS CertEd RN RM
Independent investigator and midwife, London

Six Steps to **Effective Management**

Ann Young BA MBA RGN RNT FRSH
Subject Leader, Strategic & International Management, East London
Business School, University of East London, Dagenham, Essex

Foreword

To my mind the need to find a way of understanding and communicating relatively complex ideas is itself becoming ever-more urgent; not just within the world of the moving image and the media more generally, but across the whole of our society.

Puttnam 1999

Read a selection of complaint letters to any health care organisation and somewhere, in many, will be issues which could have been quickly sorted for complainants by good communication. Ask patients, clients or their carers when they leave an outpatient or primary care appointment, or when they are told the diagnosis and treatment they will receive, what their understanding of the exchange was. Too many will have less than a clear idea. Indeed many may well be left feeling confused.

The drive towards improving the quality of the patient's journey is about improving access – giving users more choice in their care, and seeking their views in order not only to understand their needs and wants, but to refocus services to meet these. Communication has to be two-way, and listening and hearing, two very different skills, are increasingly crucial if we really are to deliver the top quality service professionals wish to be able to give.

Today's emphasis on governance, both corporate and clinical, should drive individuals and organisations to excellence. The importance of evidence based practice to managing risk, and ensuring lessons are well learned from incidents, near-misses and complaints, means that effective writing skills are essential. Poor record keeping has been a cause for concern for many years. Records must be accurate, factual, legible and succinct. They must also be readily accessible. Increasingly, patients or their carers wish to exercise their right to examine them. Records are also used both by the defence and prosecution when court cases ensue from critical incidents.

It is disappointing to see how often innovation and creative new ways to improve practice and the 'patient's journey' do not get shared across the service. This is arguably because those professionals who lead and implement improvement do not, and cannot, write papers and articles to share with others their success and lessons learned. We know that somewhere in the NHS are the answers to many of the challenges to improve quality and efficiency. Professionals, managers and others are working together to completely revise and reform services, but sharing of information is still poor.

In today's world we are bombarded by information in many formats. Soundbites, free newspapers, advertisements, emails and the Internet – communication, communication, communication. Or is it?

We all live in a fast changing world where 'instant gratification' seems to be the order of the day. This, in turn, gives many opportunities for misinformation, overload or complete misunderstanding.

Yet central to effective communication is understanding. Unless we have the skills to communicate well and appropriately with our patients; unless we really understand and respect each member of the team, and their contribution; unless we ensure clear prescriptions, reports and treatment orders, the patient will not only have a less than satisfactory outcome, but there may indeed be critical incidents which contribute to patients and clients being less safe and well than before they come into our care. Patients put their trust in us and trust that we will not harm them. When we do, it is often inferior or unsatisfactory communication which undermines the process.

The need for clear two-way communication is best evidenced by a recent, non-clinical experience of a colleague of mine. She was preparing an important presentation and asked her secretary to check that the hotel would have PowerPoint available. This was confirmed. On the day, she arrived to find the audience but, alas, no projector. On checking with the hotel reception, she was told that they did not possess a data projector. 'But my secretary checked yesterday and you said you had PowerPoint available' she said. And the response came 'Oh yes madam, we have power points in every room'! A clear case of words being said, and heard, but a complete absence of that essential ingredient for effective communication – understanding!

The promotion of more inter-professional education and learning to achieve improved team working and the development of mutual understanding and respect, can identify common values, knowledge, skills across professions and work settings and create a shared philosophy of care. Where these

Foreword

initiatives have succeeded is where there has been considerable thought and planning regarding matters of communication and language to be used, so that the experience is of value to all participants. As with patients, the use of appropriate language and terms to foster understanding rather than promoting differences is crucial. Jargon or technical terms are unhelpful as they have the potential to create a master/servant relationship, either between different professionals, or with patients.

We each have personal, and professional responsibility for the totality of the patient/client experience. That responsibility can be discomforting to some professionals, each of whom feel they do the best for patients in their care. Many of us developed in a world which was paternalistic in how we treated patients who are now increasingly better informed, and rightly more demanding of the service they consider as theirs. They are the experts in their own illness. They know the symptoms and how it affects their lives, they know the small differences, handicaps, pains and discomforts which brought them to the professional asking for help. Yet how often do professionals jump to early conclusions about diagnosis and remedies without actively listening and asking searching questions to help the patient tell their story? How often do we truly ask the carers how their loved one's behaviour, or needs, have changed?

We all need to continue to strive exponentially to improve our communication skills, with each other, with senior leaders and policy makers, with our staff across the care arena and most importantly with users of the service in order to achieve excellence.

'All professionals are conspiracies against the laity', said George Bernard Shaw.

Let us, through improving our listening and communication skills, ensure this is not so. This book will considerably help the process.

Christina Edwards

Reference

Puttnam 1999 From the Uniformed Society 1999 British Library Chadwyck-Healey Lecture, held at the British Library, Euston Road, London, 23 June 1999

Preface

In these days of increasing technological advances and organisational change the way in which we speak, write to or contact one another has become more complex and, it seems, more important to professionals providing or managing health care. Although communication has always been a key skill for the competent clinical professional, this has not automatically translated into the way these important staff members relate to others outside the direct patient relationship. The purpose of this book is to provide a range of insights into the mechanics, purpose and skills of communication to assist clinical professionals to approach their broadening remit in 'modern' health care systems. The book is part of a series which aims to inform clinical professionals about issues they need to be conversant with as their roles develop and focus less and less on direct patient care to the exclusion of all else (as was once perceived to be the case). Health care in the 21st century places many demands on all who work in the field with the result that nurses, therapists and doctors increasingly have to consider the context of care in order to provide patient services effectively.

Each chapter has been commissioned to illuminate an aspect of communication to a particular level of detail. Inevitably some chapters treat their subject in greater depth than others due to the complexity of the subject and the need to convey basic ideas as a foundation for further work by the reader. The book therefore cannot provide all the answers, nor does it seek to. Communication is by definition a complex subject and has been the focus of much research and academic discourse in recent years. Many chapters seek to provide an overview of this work where appropriate while guiding the reader to examine their skills and, where possible, to develop them. The format is designed to encourage in-depth reading, quick reference and focused learning as determined by the needs of the reader.

Each chapter has one or two 'applications' which provide either practical ways of developing skills or more detail on a facet of the subject matter of the chapter.

The book is divided into three sections. Section One covers topics relevant to personal communication aimed at identifying personal needs and ways to develop improved skills in, for example, one-to-one communication, negotiation and assertiveness. Section Two covers organisational or systems-oriented communication with particular reference to such important skills as networking, group communication and presentation. Finally Section Three examines the nature of communication in terms of specific skills (writing), tools (survey methods) or technology (email). By dividing the book in this way the editor has aimed to address what are perceived to be 'key' aspects of communication in the rapidly evolving world of health care provision.

Ultimately it is hoped that the book will provide clinical professionals with a basic toolkit and a reference work for development. The book cannot hope to provide everything the reader would wish to know on the subject but it should provide sufficient information to impress on clinicians the importance of effective communication as a basis for getting what they need to improve patient care. In the NHS of today, for example, the ability to understand the system and how to work within it depends on communicating with people who, despite working for the same organisation, do not automatically appreciate the patient perspective or clinical needs. Indeed, this may even extend to a requirement to argue a case in settings where clearly competing needs exist and where resources are limited. Without good communication skills and an appreciation of the perspective of those the clinician is seeking to influence, very little might be achieved. Put simply, it cannot be assumed that non-clinical colleagues will appreciate the best interests of patients without key elements being explained to them. The deployment of good communication skills will not guarantee success but it will improve the prospects of it.

There has been a deluge of policy initiatives (White Papers and Health Service Circulars) in the National Health Service since the Labour government was elected in 1997. This 'deluge' is likely to continue with their reelection in 2001 despite assurances that bureaucracy will be reined in during their second term of office. The fact of the matter is that politicians wish to ensure success and achievement of the targets they set for the NHS as they struggle to standardise the service and care that people can expect to receive. This places an onus on clinicians to put the arguments for the resources they need or the organisational developments required to improve the service. This will increasingly necessitate working in different environments, addressing varied audiences (including the public) and developing the ability to influence and persuade others. For some groups such as nurses and therapists this includes the need to persuade groups such as doctors or board members of the importance of developments in a particular service that might compete for resources with medicine.

Clinical governance, for example, heralds a new era for placing clinical quality at the heart of acute and primary care trust agendas. Do non-doctors feel equipped to put the case for ensuring that 'clinical' means more than medicine? This book should provide the impetus to non-medical clinicians to develop the skills and knowledge they need to make sure that clinical governance impacts on all aspects of the clinical service, as is intended by the government. Communication skills lie at the heart of this. It is interesting to note that with recent criticism of the medical profession, prompted by a number of high-profile clinical scandals, and the proposed reform of the General Medical Council, it could be suggested that there is much many doctors could learn from a book of this nature!

If you recognise a need to develop your communication skills this book will set you off on a journey that should prove very rewarding personally, professionally and clinically.

Shoreham-by-Sea   Mark Darley
2001

Section **One**

PERSONAL COMMUNICATION

OVERVIEW

This section deals with aspects of communication which either impact directly on the individual or which depend on the development of personal skills. The four chapters are intended to build on the awareness and insight developed from a deeper understanding of, in the first instance, assertiveness so that the nurse manager or health care professional can approach communication confidently. This also provides the practitioner with coping mechanisms for situations when things do not go to plan or a challenge is evident. It is important to remember that in communicating with colleagues within the health care setting or with people from outside, many outcomes cannot be predicted. This is particularly so when dealing with reactions to things said, done or required that demand a difficult decision to be made or which prompt heated debate and discussion.

This book, by its very existence, suggests that communication and associated skills are not only important in themselves but that they are important to health care professionals and nurses wishing to maximise their impact in management settings within the National Health Service. Knowing how to handle one-to-one communication and what influences successful outcomes will help get desired results, earn respect from management peers and others and provide a foundation for renewed professional confidence in a rapidly changing clinical world.

A step on from learning effective one-to-one communication is the skill of negotiation and how, if this is done well, this can contribute to the achievement of goals. Communication is not, as the book demonstrates, a simple affair and negotiation will be a regular feature of life for nurse managers and other clinical professionals with responsibility for patient/client groups or resources. Nothing is given easily in a world where competing demands for resources suggest that every service development or change will be achieved through hard work and arguing the case above the merits of others. Learning to negotiate will become a required skill in these situations.

Finally, some thoughts and insights are provided on the thinking behind marketing yourself as a means of illustrating how the perceptions of nurses influence the way they are received in, for example, management circles. Understanding this prepares the nurse manager in particular for a range of reactions to their involvement in management matters. Despite progress in recent years, where examples of nurses acting as effective and respected NHS managers have proliferated, it is not always the case that others, especially non-clinical managers, will accept nurses in this type of role. Effective self-marketing is intended to assist the aspiring nurse manager to develop ways of overcoming such potential barriers.

'Applications', used to illustrate key themes or points raised in the main text, complete each chapter. Taken together, the knowledge, skills and practical advice contained in the first four chapters of the book provide a solid foundation for improved management practice as well as a prompt for further study.

Chapter **One**

Assertiveness

Colleen Wedderburn Tate

- Definitions
- Respect for others
- Respect for yourself
- Self-awareness
- Effective, clear and consistent communication

- Transactional analysis
- Life positions
- Assertiveness, aggression or passivity
- Assertiveness in action
- The 10/10 exercise

OVERVIEW

To be assertive is to communicate in a particular way. Whether at home, at work or in social settings, knowing when and how to act assertively is a key communication, as well as a social, skill. This chapter offers practical information about being assertive, as well as practical solutions to enhance your ability to be assertive, with particular reference to health care. The Applications section of the chapter focuses on techniques to remove barriers to behaving assertively and ends with an exercise to promote familiarity and ease with the key elements of assertiveness.

INTRODUCTION

I own a T-shirt on which is printed: *I suppose you want me to be assertive. Well, I'm not going to be OK.* What was your first reaction on reading that? Depending where you place the punctuation marks, the statement can be read negatively (as written) or positively (a comma before OK). Is this a statement of assertion? I will come back to this phrase later on.

DEFINITIONS

To assert is to 'declare; state clearly; insist on one's rights or opinions; demand recognition'. To be assertive is to 'assert oneself; positive, forthright'. It can also be defined as 'dogmatic', meaning imposing personal opinions or being arrogant. To be described as dogmatic can be a grievous insult and fear of this is an excellent barrier to behaving assertively. Yet, as part of communication, assertive behaviour consists of imparting feelings, emotions and opinions. At issue is how we do this effectively without denying ourselves, and others, the right to express freely. In health care settings, assertive behaviour is a key element in ensuring that patient care is delivered appropriately. Yet, as many nurses can testify, being assertive is sometimes seen as 'not knowing your place'. The events arising from the enquiry into the postoperative paediatric deaths at Bristol Royal Infirmary would seem to indicate that for some doctors, an assertive nurse is a liability and should not be permitted to challenge clinical judgement (Davidson 1998). Nurses, being primarily women, also seem to display ambivalence about assertiveness, often preferring to act passively even when this is not appropriate.

But why do we need to be assertive? Think about the key communication skills listed below.

- Planning and preparing
- Listening and observing
- Assessment and decision making
- Questioning and probing
- Giving feedback
- Reflection and evaluation

All these skills require the ability to establish communication, maintain it and review it. All these skills are needed for the effective delivery of patient care. To complete the communicate/maintain/review cycle, you experience vulnerability, criticism, hostility and success. Your assertive sense is needed to meet all these challenges and help others (both colleagues and patients) meet theirs. It is not possible to communicate effectively if what we want to say is artificially suppressed by fear, anger or other barriers. Additionally, communication can be stressful. Assertive behaviour is a positive response to stress and can prevent some of the physiological consequences generated by negative responses to stress.

Therefore, you could say that assertiveness is a *communication style*, just as shouting, aggression, passivity, bullying, crying, sulking and smiling are. The issue is less one of 'good or bad' styles (although I would say that bullying is not a helpful communication style in the long term) but rather, what is an appropriate response to an event. An assertive communication style can be as out of place as aggression or passivity. For example, forcing someone to be assertive is close to bullying. On the other hand, expressing your strong opinions in such a way that others are offended and then refusing to accept their right to be offended is not assertiveness. Assertiveness comprises:

- respect for other people
- respect for yourself (or self-esteem)
- self-awareness
- effective, clear and consistent communication.

Let us look at each of these individual elements.

RESPECT FOR OTHERS

Respect for others means that we respect their right to make demands, ask favours and express their feelings. When we respect others they are more likely to use appropriate behaviours in responding to our demands, feelings and needs. In my clinical practice as a midwife, respecting the wishes of pregnant women is the basis of a happy birth experience. This does not mean that women get exactly what they want. Part of respecting others is to speak the truth as you know it. For example, if a pregnant woman demands a caesarean section for delivery, I must express my knowledge of the risks she and her baby face from this procedure. My aim is not to discourage her intention but to inform it. Recent cases of women being 'forced' to have caesarean sections against their expressed wishes may be one result of a failure of communication between the woman and her carers and a lack of listening to each other's needs and feelings.

RESPECT FOR YOURSELF (SELF-ESTEEM)

Having respect for yourself makes you less likely to be dependent on other people for approval and self-worth and less likely to act against your will. This can prevent you from following a course of action that you know to be wrong or inappropriate. It is not necessary to look to the Nuremberg trials to find examples of people who claim that others made them act in a certain way. No-one can *make* you do anything against your will, unless you choose to accept that another person can control your thoughts and actions. (An exception may be coercion by physical force or torture, but such circumstances are relatively unusual and not always successful.) Having self-respect enables us to withstand such pressure, to recover more quickly from mishaps and use these experiences as opportunities for learning.

SELF-AWARENESS

Self-awareness enables you to approach every circumstance with some idea of what might happen and how you might feel about it. This way, we can take responsibility for our emotions and are less likely to blame others if events do not turn out the way we thought they would. For example, the impact of general management and the 1991 reforms left many health care professionals at that time struggling to find an effective role in the planning and development of health care. In particular, many health care managers appeared not to value the contribution of nursing or other non-medical clinical professionals to health care planning and delivery. For their part, many health care professionals (nurses in particular) have difficulty in articulating their contribution and feel that they lack influence (Smith 1998). Even directors of nursing appeared frustrated by their inability to convince non-nurse directors of the importance of nursing (Girvan 1998). Generally, health care professionals were slow to recognise the impact that changes in health care provision and management would have on their role. The traditional approach, that the health service could not do without their services, has blinded many to the need for a reassessment of what they do and how it is done. Self-awareness is a function of self-esteem. A flaw in one can distort the other.

Personal communication

EFFECTIVE, CLEAR AND CONSISTENT COMMUNICATION

Effective communication ensures that others understand what we say and what we mean. It also ensures that they know that we understand what they want from us. Communicating in clear and consistent ways means that we are less likely to mislead, mystify and maltreat others and even ourselves.

Central to the four elements of assertiveness is how we express our assertiveness, especially in speech. We can use words to stroke as well as to strike. Because communicating is like acting in a play (everyone has a script of some kind, either shared or secret), the words we say and the behavioural response we get to what we say can provide signals about how much of our real selves will be welcomed on stage. The following example illustrates this. When we meet a person for the first time, one of the key interactions is finding ways to observe the social conventions. Do not, for example, stare or smile too much or too often; concentrate on what the other person is saying; do not spit; do not drop ash on their exposed skin. This intricate ballet offers many opportunities for comedy, if the results were not so often painful. Long before we meet a person we have decided how we will deal with them (or communicate). This is the realm of transactional analysis.

TRANSACTIONAL ANALYSIS

Transactional analysis (or TA) has developed exponentially since first introduced by Eric Berne in his books *Games people play* (Berne 1968) and *What do you say after you say hello?* (Berne 1975). The underlying philosophy is summed up in the title of a book by Thomas Harris (1973): *I'm OK, you're OK*. This phrase has come to mean 'win-win', the idea that all of us have intrinsic value, that we act in ways which enable us to get on with others and that we have the right to have our needs met. Because TA encompasses this 'win-win' belief system, issues of assertiveness and autonomy are a key feature. We all come to every interaction with attitudes (beliefs, emotions, fears and behaviour) which are either open to change or serve to reinforce our view of the world. Because few of these attitudes are available for close inspection, we focus on what is visible – the behaviour.

So, you meet a new colleague who talks fast and furious. As you only ever meet this person in settings where they are talking, your view of them will be very different from someone else who sees them dealing with bereaved relatives. Your beliefs about people who talk fast will be reinforced by their behaviour, leading you to perceive them only as a fast talker. Such attitude labelling can have serious consequences: we see one part of a person and assume that that is their whole being. The power of transactional analysis is to enable us to break this tendency to label and see the world as it is.

LIFE POSITIONS

'Win-win' is one of the four life positions described below. Power and feelings of powerlessness are implicit in these life positions and therefore in debates about assertiveness. Inevitably, gender becomes an issue because women generally feel and act powerless, especially at work, while men may feel powerless but act powerful (which gives the aura of power). The behaviour we choose in any given circumstance depends on whether we perceive the world as frightening, friendly or full of harm.

The four main life positions, with examples, are outlined below.

1. I'm OK, you're not OK (putting people down because you think you are smarter than them at all times; manipulative; aggressive).
2. You're OK, I'm not OK (unable to make decisions; being envious of another's life; passive).
3. I'm not OK, you're not OK (complaining about misfortune, especially with others of like mind; passive/aggressive).
4. I'm OK, you're OK (accepting, tolerant, assertive).

It is at this fourth life position that we should aim to spend the majority of our time.

The other three positions are options we choose from when, for whatever reason, the world bites back. They are behaviours which you may recognise from theories of how we respond to stress: we fight (aggressive) or we flee (passive). Choosing to act assertively is both a behavioural style and a communication style. Fight and flight are both appropriate behaviours. However, when we are assertive, aggression and passivity are less likely to be reflex actions or random behaviours. In other words, being assertive gives you control over your behaviour and therefore over how other people respond to you. But how do we decide when to be assertive, aggressive or passive?

Personal communication

ASSERTIVE, AGGRESSIVE OR PASSIVE?

We tend to choose our behaviours based on previous experience. An example might be as follows. At a party you meet a blue-eyed person. You are happy because you always get on with blue-eyed people; they always smile back and know how to have fun. At the same party you are introduced to a green-eyed person and you wish they would go away. You have never liked such people; they are cold, censorious killjoys. How did you come to these conclusions about people based solely on eye colour? Is this attitude labelling? We all tend to see only what we expect to see. Blue-eyed people are perceived as warm because we treat them that way and they respond accordingly. Green-eyed people are cold to us because they are responding to our coldness to them. So we reinforce each other's behaviour, for good or ill. (Of course, an assertive green-eyed person would probably accept that you are just having an off day, not indulging in random behaviour!) Choosing whether to be assertive, aggressive or passive depends on the results we expect to get or that we received in the past. Consider the following situations and decide on a suitable response – aggressive, assertive or passive.

- A friend asks to borrow money, which is a regular event. This time you cannot really afford to help as you are saving up for a weekend trip. She says that if you do not lend her the money she will have to get it 'by other means'.
- Three months ago you requested a particular day off for a special occasion. However, you now see that other people who made their requests later have got what they want but you have not.
- Someone you work with has a reputation for being 'difficult'. On the rota you notice that you will be working with this person on every shift for the next 7 days. You have heard rumours that this person is lazy and not particularly good at their job. On your first shift together she is over 20 minutes late.
- At lunch one day a colleague from another department complains about the behaviour of another colleague whom you consider to be a friend. He asks you to tell your friend how angry he is feeling.
- You stay in all day and the TV repair company does not turn up as agreed.

How you respond to any of these events depends on how you perceive yourself in relation to the people making requests of you,

Assertiveness

your assumptions about how they will respond to your response and your notions of power. Almost all communications are requests of one kind or another – mostly to be listened to. Furthermore, all communications have implicit power relationships. If you perceive others as more powerful than you, then you are more likely to respond passively, usually by doing something you do not want to. Conversely, if you perceive that you are more powerful than others, you are more likely to display manipulative behaviour.

Perceiving power as an attribute possessed by everyone is more likely to trigger assertive behaviours but, depending on the level of threat we perceive in an encounter, we can, and do, adapt our behaviour. Phrases such as 'the worm turned', 'the straw that broke the camel's back' and 'enough is enough' are evidence that, given a high enough level of threat to self, we behave differently. Unfortunately, this often means going from passive to aggressive, without stopping at assertive. The gender and cultural undertones in aggression, passivity and assertiveness tend to complicate the issue.

In most societies, power is concomitant with authority. Most of the images we have of this relate to men and many are modelled on military styles of command and authority. In contrast, one of the few images of authority related to women is that of the mother. As the predominant arena of men is the public domain and that of the mother is the private world of the home (with its notions of peace, calm and comfort), there is a tendency to equate passive actions with women and aggressive actions with men. Even when women hold positions of authority, aggressive behaviour is derided. Consider the image of Margaret Thatcher subduing recalcitrant Cabinet ministers with her metaphorical handbag. Hardly a positive image of a powerful woman.

In her book *Talking from 9–5*, Deborah Tannen (1995) argues that generally, men come with the image of authority; that is, physical appearance – body size, height, voice. But this association of authority with maleness also pervades our language. Tannen gives the example of Japanese 'particles' – little words that have no real meaning but give emphasis to sentences (comparable 'particles' in English are 'right', 'isn't it?', 'OK?'). In Japan men and women apparently use different particles and men will use female particles when speaking to women in order to appear less authoritarian and male ones for the opposite effect (Tannen 1995).

Hence, being female is associated with soft, non-threatening words – polite, submissive, gentle, mild. Therefore women who want to be more authoritative risk being viewed as male. Probably the only exception to this is when a woman is protecting her children. Then, she assumes a more male role *for another, but not for herself.* The prevailing stereotypes of authoritative women as bitches, witches or whores are detrimental for both men and women, in the public as well as the private sphere. Denying anyone their right to full self-expression creates a perfect climate for miscommunication, confusion and, ultimately, dysfunctional behaviour. But assertive behaviour appears to be easier to achieve, and more acceptable, in some settings than in others.

ASSERTIVENESS IN ACTION

At work

For many of us, being assertive at work is relatively easy. Especially in health care, our rules for professional conduct legitimise the challenges we make to each other in pursuit of high-quality patient care or to improve practice. Although, as seemingly in the Bristol case, another professional may not accept our right to challenge, we are less afraid of challenging people in authority because there are codes to back us up. Nurses in particular are aware of the penalties of breaching the UKCC Code of Conduct. Assertive nurses will raise the hackles of those who equate 'nurse' with 'soft and not very bright'. Few managers or doctors now overtly suggest that a nurse's place is by the bedside but from personal experience, assertive behaviour at work remains difficult to use, as the following example shows.

One of my professional experiences included a situation where a consultant refused to do ward rounds with anyone except the blue-dressed senior midwife in overall charge of the ward on the day of the round. A primary midwifery pilot scheme had been created on the ward with the purpose of giving midwives more professional autonomy over the care they provided. Midwives in the pilot gave total care to groups of 5–7 women as part of a 'practice make-over' in this women's health unit (including gynaecology). The traditional ward round was now therefore inappropriate as a method of reviewing care. Prior to commencing the pilot, I met ward staff and talked at length about the purpose of primary nursing and midwifery with all the consultants. They had all seemed enthusiastic and supportive of the need to create a more personalised and humane way of delivering care. However, I was surprised when staff refused to perform ward rounds. The consultant involved confronted me with the accusation of disrupting patient

Assertiveness

care for no good reason, of creating confusion by not having 'a blue dress' lead the ward round and demanded to know what I was going to do about it. I agreed to find a solution within 48 hours.

The next day I met the consultant by accident and said that I had found a solution to the problem: from now on, all midwives will wear grey. This was, of course, premised on the assertion that the midwife's skill and knowledge, rather than the uniform, are the important factors in a ward round.

Some readers might think that my suggested solution was flippant, discourteous or even rude. My aim was twofold: respect the consultant's right to make the request and disarm the conflict. Well-placed humour is only one way of doing this, based on your judgement of the importance of the issue under discussion. To my mind, the colour of the uniform was of far less importance than the intelligence and skills of the person wearing the uniform. Furthermore, it is difficult to argue with the truth. Was the consultant really saying that the colour of the dress was more important than the ability to provide information about patient care? Unlikely. So why make mountains out of molehills? The pilot was successful. The relevance of traditional uniform was answered when, as a result of developing a woman-centred service, all midwives in the unit adopted a new uniform – navy skirt or slacks and white shirts.

The story related above is mild in comparison to what, no doubt, other health care workers have experienced. Nursing, a profession still adhering to a hierarchy, has only recently begun to feel comfortable with 'assertive' behaviour among its practitioners. Probably the biggest boost to this is the removal of student nurse training from hospitals to mainstream higher education. This is not to deny that universities have their problems with issues of assertiveness, but nursing's removal from the strait-jacket of a system modelled on Victorian households, namely hospitals, has freed nurses from the passivity and submissiveness which have been a marked feature of our history. But nurses, along with other health care professionals, still work within organisations which are hierarchical, containing some people who would prefer us to remain passive.

We still have to negotiate on what is appropriate behaviour for women and for men who are not part of a dominant profession. That has not, does not and will not stop health care staff being assertive where it is needed, especially when attempting to define what nursing and health care is and is not.

Keyzer (1988) tells a story about the implementation of the nursing process (at the time, a new form of documenting care) in a health authority which illustrates where we need to target our energies if we are to get rewards from being assertive.

The health authority was keen to implement the nursing process and the chosen area was care of the elderly. The medically dominated, high-technology wards were not included. Part of the implementation of the nursing process is the redefinition of what nurses do and what nursing is – the nurse as a planner and giver of care and an autonomous practitioner. Yet a patient information handout from a community hospital in this health authority described doctors as the ones who cared for the patient and controlled access to other caregivers. The nurse's role was perceived to be more that of liaison – keeping in touch with other caregivers and ensuring that patients received the care they needed. In other words, the traditional view of nurses as passive doers was preferred to the equal partner in giving care which is explicit in the nursing process.

These perceptions persist. Unfortunately, some nurses aid these perceptions, especially when they fail to assert their contribution to policy making, general management and the wider arena of health politics. For nurses to assert themselves at work, in the face of prevailing stereotypes, they have to believe in all four pillars of assertive behaviour, not just the first one.

- Respect other people
- Respect for yourself (or self-esteem)
- Self-awareness
- Effective, clear and consistent communication

The same applies to being assertive at home.

At home

If some talk shows are to be believed, all over the world women and men are preventing each other from being assertive at home. The men who choose their wives' clothes, friends and food; the wives who will not let their husbands go out with their male friends. People who appear on talk shows to parade the mess that is their life may indeed need therapy but they are telling us something about how social norms operate in the private sphere of the home. They are also using the medium which more than ever gives strong signals about the consequences that women suffer when they behave assertively – usually by losing a man of immense wealth and power. One message seems to be clear: it is OK to rule the office but leave that sort of thing at the front door when you come home.

Assertiveness

At home, assertive behaviour does create problems, especially for women. As men's roles become less clear and uncertain, some act out their authority needs in what has traditionally been the woman's sphere – the home. If the woman is an authority figure at work, she is likely to bring some of that into the home, creating tension and conflict with partner, parents and children. For example, ordering food in a restaurant or hailing a taxi on the street, common occurrences for many working women, can be seen by men as treading on their territory. On the other hand, if you behave like a doormat at home, that also causes problems.

Assertiveness is based on equality – the equal right to express feelings, make demands and respect others and yourself. But, even after several decades of feminism and a few years of the 'new man', many men, and some women, equate equality with dominance. This perception also applies to people from ethnic minorities who are often accused of being aggressive when acting assertively. Hence the difficulty many organizations have with reducing discriminatory practices. Making a demand for equality is often taken as making a demand to be dominant. Tannen (1995) argues that such perceptions operate on the assumption that every relationship is hierarchical, with a boss (dominant) role and a subordinate. If this assumption is held to be true, then if the people who traditionally have been allocated the role of subordinate – women, children, elderly people, black people, disabled people – refuse to accept the role, then they must want to take the dominant/boss role (Tannen 1995). One way of clarifying this confusion is to be clear in your own mind about what assertive behaviour is and communicate this to others.

THE 10/10 EXERCISE

As a means of developing your own thoughts on this, why not try the 10/10 exercise. This can be done at the end of the day, helping you to clear your head, with the advantage of being done at home with the people you live with. The purpose of the exercise is to give each person 10 minutes of unconditional listening time, preferably daily but if not, at least twice each week. There are six ground rules for this exercise.

1. Choose a time when you will all be in the house together. If this is not possible for someone, have them choose a listener with whom they will do the exercise at an agreed time.
2. Everyone has 10 minutes to talk about anything they want to. What is not permitted is to verbally attack the other people involved in the exercise. (That is for another time.)

3. The listener(s) will make no comments, suggestions or other-wise interrupt the speaker.
4. When everyone has spoken, people can then make requests of each other for help, support or advice.
5. At the end of the process, agree the next meeting, and say 'thank you'.
6. Between sessions, feelings or information must not be used to judge or otherwise malign the speaker.

When you first try this exercise, beware of the following.

● Many people find active listening threatening, partly because of the undivided attention but mostly because it so rarely happens that we do not know how to do it.
● Active listening is very hard work. We are more used to telling than listening.
● Making requests for help or support may also seem threatening, with its overtones of not being able to cope or being incompe-tent.
● Active listening requires practice, consistently.
● The ground rules must be used to prevent the exercise being an excuse for emotional abuse.

The value of this exercise is threefold.

1. People get undivided attention (that is, positive strokes).
2. We learn how to listen.
3. We remember to say 'thank you'.

Much of what passes for communication between people is really wrestling with your words for room to manoeuvre. By doing the 10/10 exercise, we all get to speak about issues that are of concern to us, without interruption or lack of concentration of the listener.

CONCLUSION

As has been made clear in this chapter, the four components of assertive behaviour are respect for other people, respect for yourself (or self-esteem), self-awareness and effective, clear and consistent communication. Although the concept of assertiveness can be viewed negatively, I hope I have shown in this chapter how this 'perception' can be turned around and made to work for you if you so wish. The Application section at the end of the chapter goes over some of the material again to reinforce practical things you can do to be assertive in your work and communication and therefore more effective.

Assertiveness

Personal communication

Practice checklist

- Plan for your next attendance at a meeting where you usually experience conflict or feel you don't get a chance to have your say. Plan to include accepting that conflict exists, listening openly and suspending whatever is your usual behaviour in the meeting. Rehearse what you want to say and ask for the agenda.
- Practise self-awareness – actively listen to the words you use when you're feeling threatened or unsure of yourself. Be more aware of your body language (non-verbal communication is often more powerful than what you say), eye contact, the pitch of your voice (when we're scared or unsure, our voice rises in pitch because we aren't breathing properly).
- Use the 10/10 exercise outlined on p. 14 – after you've clearly communicated with the other person involved what you want to do and why!

References

Berne E 1968 Games people play. Penguin, Harmondsworth

Berne E 1975 What do you say after you say hello? Corgi, London

Davidson L 1998 Alarm unheard or unheeded? Health Service Journal 108(5607): 14–15

Girvan J 1998 Satisfaction and motivation. Nursing Management 5(4): 11–15

Harris T 1973 I'm OK, you're OK. Pan, Harmondsworth

Keyzer D 1988 Challenging role boundaries: conceptual frameworks for understanding the conflict arising from the implementation of the nursing process in practice. In: White R (ed) Political issues in nursing, vol 3. Wiley, Chichester

Smith F 1998 Children's services: why managers lack power. Nursing Management 5(4): 6–7

Tannen D 1995 Talking from 9–5: how women's and men's conversational styles affect who gets ahead, who gets heard, who gets credit, and what gets done at work. Virago, London

Further reading

Burnard P 1992 Assertiveness skills. In: Effective communication skills for health professionals. Chapman and Hall, London

Duck S 1985 Social and personal relationships. In: Knapp MI, Miller GR (eds) Handbook of interpersonal communication. Sage, Beverly Hills, California

Goffman E 1971 The presentation of self in everyday life. Penguin, Harmondsworth

Hay J 1993 Working it out at work: understanding attitudes and building relationships. Sherwood Publishing, Watford
In this book, Julie Hay uses transactional analysis as the basis for some self-awareness activities that can help to break lifelong habits which inhibit the way we think, behave and feel.

Mendell A 1996 How men think: the seven essential rules for making it in a man's world. Fawcett/Columbine, New York
Adrienne Mendell presents some intriguing findings from her interviews with 100 male executives and from counselling career women. For example, when a woman apologises for making a mistake, men think she is admitting to being incompetent.

Shea M 1994 Personal impact: the art of good communication. Mandarin, London
A neat little book from a writer with a public relations background.

Tannen D 1992 You just don't understand *and* That's not what I meant. Virago, London
Deborah Tannen is a linguist (i.e. she studies the science of language and its structure) who has written many popular books on communication.

Walmsley C 1993 Assertiveness: the right to be you. BBC Books, London
This is a pocket-sized handbook on assertiveness and is very user friendly.

Assertiveness

Application 1:1
Colleen Wedderburn Tate

Barriers to behaving assertively

Listed below for ease of reference are some of the barriers to assertiveness. Do you accept all of these or do some not apply to you and your working experience? Can you add to the list?

Write down what the 'fear of rejection', means to you. Is this a legitimate fear and how do you think it manifests itself in your attempts to be more assertive? Once you have been through all the barriers you recognise and made notes of how these impact on you, devise an action plan to remedy the most critical factors. If you have a mentor or clinical supervisor you may wish to use this rough exercise to gain another person's view of the points you have made. This is a safe environment in which to do this and it may even make you aware of issues you had not considered or allay your concerns in other areas.

- Fear of rejection
- Previous bad experience
- Fear of failing
- Fear of upsetting people
- Other people's perceptions
- Self-perception
- Fear of retaliation
- Lack of knowledge and skills
- Emotional problems
- Psychological problems
- Fear of losing control
- Lack of self-esteem
- Lack of self-confidence
- Lack of support for change in behaviour
- Fear of other people's response
- Fear of change
- Unwillingness to change
- Incomplete understanding of the term 'assertiveness'

- Lack of role models
- Feelings of powerlessness
- Gender and cultural issues

Assertiveness is important for people to get their point across and to contribute fully in the work environment. If used well, a new approach to assertiveness can bring untold benefits to you and those you work with or care for.

THE THINGS PEOPLE SAY

The following is a list of actual reasons I have been given for a reluctance to behave assertively. Do you recognise any of them?

1. I will upset people.
2. People will not like me.
3. I would have to be more aggressive.
4. It is unfeminine.
5. I might lose my temper.
6. I might make people cry.
7. People might think I am aggressive.
8. My friends will not like it.
9. I will feel uncomfortable.
10. I will get a bad report from my boss.
11. My staff will complain.
12. People will laugh at me.
13. They will not believe me.
14. I will have to be different.
15. I will feel stupid.
16. I am too young.
17. Men will not like it.
18. I will not know what to say.
19. I will not get promoted.
20. My boss would not like it.
21. I am not like that.
22. I would not know how to do it.
23. It is too American.
24. I am too small (physically).
25. My voice is too soft.
26. It did not work when I tried it.
27. When I try I always fail.
28. It does not work.
29. My mother/friends/family would stop loving me.
30. It is too difficult.

Barriers to behaving assertively

PRACTISING GETTING IT RIGHT

This is a simple exercise designed to make you comfortable with the four elements.

1. Write out the four components of assertive behaviour (see Chapter 1). Tape them to a board or surface that you have to look at at least once a day and say them out loud as often as possible.
Rationale: The more you say something, the more you believe it.

2. Stand in a front of a mirror, put your hand at the bottom of your rib cage (where your diaphragm is) and breathe in. Breathe out. Do this sequence five or six times until you get accustomed to how you feel when you breathe properly. (Warning: the first few times you might feel light-headed so keep a chair or support close by.)
Rationale: Incorrect breathing detracts from your ability to speak clearly (the voice sounds thin, high and strangulated) and from what you say. Correct breathing deepens the voice. It also enables the voice to travel further and gives it more authority.

3. Say the words 'I want' three times, First, emphasise the 'I', then the 'want'. Then say the phrase with even emphasis. Do you notice any difference in the tone of your voice each time?
Rationale: When speaking assertively, equal emphasis is given to all words. This does not mean monotonic speech or speaking without emphasis, but emphasis is used appropriately and in the right places.

4. If you have difficulty saying 'no', practise in front of a mirror for as long as it takes to feel silly.
Rationale: The face moves in weird lines when mouthing the word 'no'. By noticing, and laughing at, this, when you have to tell someone 'no', you will start to smile at this memory. Your voice therefore sounds less tight and less guilty (if this is one of your panic buttons).

5. Practise slumping (head down, shoulders rounded, chin tucked in to chest) while saying 'I want to discuss a pay rise'.
Rationale: Slumping makes it difficult to breathe appropriately and therefore to use the full power of your voice. If this sounds obvious, freeze your position now. How are you sitting or standing?

6. Use more proactive (precise) words, and fewer reactive (imprecise) ones. For example, if you tend to use the word 'nice' to indicate feeling, start saying precisely what you are feeling. If you are asked how you are, describe it precisely, rather than saying 'I am fine'.
Rationale: If the other person is really interested and not just being polite, they will actively listen to you instead of glazing over.

7. If you know you need to be assertive over a particular issue, wear something that makes you feel really good (clothes, jewellery, hair style, make-up).
Rationale: If you feel good, you will act more confidently.

8. Use simple words, and say exactly what you mean.
Rationale: The simpler the words, the less the confusion. When you speak plainly, there is less chance of you being misunderstood.

9. Always engage the brain before opening the mouth.
Rationale: If you think before you speak, you are more likely to say what you mean.

10. Pay yourself compliments.
Rationale: Behaving assertively includes thinking about yourself more, which makes you feel good about yourself, which makes you more confident, which leads to more assertive behaviour.

Behaving assertively is a communication style. It enables you to meet your own needs without interfering with other people's right to meet theirs. Behaving aggressively or passively are other types of communication which, by behaving assertively, you can choose to use more appropriately. Barriers to behaving assertively are founded in our perception of ourselves as powerless and unable to make legitimate demands for a range of needs. By removing these barriers we have the opportunity of communicating more effectively and purposefully at work, in the home and with the world at large.

Barriers to behaving assertively

Application 1:2
Ann P Young

The importance of packaging

Psychologists have long had evidence of the strong impact of image in attracting people to both things and other people and the packaging of the message is usually more influential than the content of the message (Argyle 1988).

Health care professionals need to be aware of their own individual image. Whether as practitioners or managers, they are a visible part of the team and their image is a component of the relationship they build, not only with their patients or clients but also with their work colleagues and managers (Young 1995). For example, the issue of whether to wear uniforms or not in a variety of settings can have a strong impact on the observer's view of nurses in relation to their efficiency, authority or accessibility. The implications of such decisions may be much greater than realised and health care professionals must see personal presentation as an important part of the total package that they present.

Consider the following comments from a matron of a private hospital. The private sector has long recognised the importance of image in both selling services and attracting the best medical consultants and staff to work within its organisations. The powerful effect of appearance is underlined by her words.

> I wore uniform when I was first matron and the patients and consultants loved it. They said that it signified the word matron, which is rubbish as I see hardly any patients now – unfortunately. I see them if they are very sick, I want to satisfy myself that we are providing the equipment that the nurses need, that the right people are on duty at the time, so I go to see the patient but it is for different reasons. I never go round just to say hello.
>
> About 7 years ago now, I stopped wearing uniform. It really seemed inappropriate. I started going out and lecturing to ladies' clubs and other venues to talk about the private sector. Within the hospital, I sit on the medical advisory and ethical committee, the only woman among 13 or 14 pretty powerful men. When I wore uniform, I felt they were fairly patronising, very sweet, I felt they

wanted to pat me on my frilly little hat, you pop off now, little nurse, and leave the big boys to talk about the problems. When I wore a business suit, they were horrible to me: we will not . . . lots of finger shaking, I didn't like that at all. Now I can manipulate them by appearing sort of reasonably professional, perhaps a little softer than in my power-dressed suits. And it's fine. And I now sit right next to those people who I know are going to be aggressive or have got a problem; it's difficult to lose your temper when you have someone sitting 4 inches away from you, it's quite safe if they are right over there. So I play that sort of game.

But I have changed my dress as well. At one time, it was a bit like a uniform, looked rather strict, always navy blue or black, it really looked quite the business. I don't need to do that now. I like to dress properly, the company actually pay for my clothing allowance, £500 a year which is very nice, but with that is the implication that it is all image, isn't it? Inherent in the job descriptions is the message, thou shalt not let the company down, thou shalt project the image that the company wish to be projected. We have uniform codes for everyone – and they are enforced, I enforce them. . . . it is about customer expectations and they are the ones paying. I mean, I don't agree with picking the whitest, most beautiful, with the prettiest smile, receptionists. I think that is horrible, but I do go for people who have a nice open personality and who have a winning smile, because that is my front desk, the shop window.

Her perceptions are, of course, strongly coloured by her gender (female), ethnicity (white) and the strong profit orientation of her organisation. It might be interesting to consider how a male or a non-white female manager would use appearance in similar circumstances.

However, no professional in any setting can avoid the issue of image. It is important and has a strong influence on how we relate to others, whether they are external clients or internal colleagues. Quality management views all these people as customers and certainly such thinking was very apparent from this particular matron.

Now spend some time considering the effect, firstly that others' appearance has on you, and then, that your appearance has on others. List some negative and positive points for each category. Decide what image you consider it is important to project and why. How do you go about achieving this? What about influencing others? Uniform policies are notoriously difficult to uphold. If you consider appearance as part of the image projected by your particular professional group, how can you encourage involvement and compliance?

A conclusion is that individual health care professionals should be clear on what, in their view, it is important to portray. Ideally, they should participate in decisions concerning this matter in order to promote the commitment necessary for an organisation to develop its own particular 'brand' image.

The importance of packaging

References

Argyle M 1988 Bodily communication, 2nd edn. Routledge, London

Young AP 1995 Is marketing an obligatory skill in the nursing role? British Journal of Nursing 4(16): 965–968

Personal communication

Chapter **Two**

One-to-one communication

Mark Darley, Fiona McGreuer

- ● **What is one-to-one communication?**
- ● **The clinical professional as communicator**
- ● **The role of the senses in communication**
- ● **Working relationships**

- ● **Stress levels and communication**
- ● **Models of communication**
- ● **Composition of a message**
- ● **Elements of a message**
- ● **Listening**

OVERVIEW

This chapter provides a basic analysis of an important aspect of personal communication: one-to-one communication. While many people think that such communication is largely a matter of words and what you say, this is not so. The chapter discusses appearance, body language and other issues which influence the ability of an individual to communicate effectively in face-to-face situations. Finally, the critical skill of listening is discussed as a means of showing that communication is a two-way process and not limited to what an individual may want to say. The overriding impression therefore is that direct communication with another person is far more complex than most of us think. It is hoped that this chapter will shed a little light on the subject and encourage the reader to explore in detail the concepts outlined here.

INTRODUCTION

One-to-one communication or how we relate to one another directly is an important aspect of an understanding of communication. This chapter will examine the elements of communication between people in order to give the reader a framework for understanding this vital aspect of practice. This is important in direct patient or client contact, as might be expected, but it is in the wider arena that these skills become crucial to the clinical professional, notably, for example, in putting the case for more resources or explaining an aspect of clinical practice to non-clinical colleagues.

An interesting article by Lloyd (1994) looked at communication in trusts and other health care organisations. It examined methods of communicating and researched trust and health authority internal and external communications objectives. Its findings were that priorities tended to focus on the following.

- Internal matters
  1. Ensuring staff understood the goals and objectives of the organisation
  2. Promoting identity and commitment to the organisation and encouraging team working and a sense of belonging
  3. Consulting staff and providing opportunities for them to express their views and ideas
  4. Keeping staff informed of developments
- External matters
  1. Receiving feedback from patients
  2. Building a strong image and identity (of the organisation)
  3. Providing information
  4. Promoting understanding of the organisation's aims

All these objectives are very laudable and pertinent for health service organisations but it is noticeable that they concentrate on outcomes rather than the process or 'how to' communicate. Lloyd concluded that the crucial issue was that the communication skills of managers were often insufficiently developed to ensure that these managerially focused priorities were properly understood.

Although health care professionals might consider their own communication skills to be well developed, this cannot be taken for granted. What follows attempts to provide basic insight into the key elements of one-to-one communication to ensure that when clinicians function in areas outside the clinical setting they do not repeat the failures that seem to have been identified by Lloyd.

Personal communication

Although one-to-one communication relies to a great extent on interpersonal contact and skills, the increasingly technical nature of many forms of modern communication can persuade some managers that this is the best way to communicate in the health services of today. While such things as email, fax and video conferencing speed up communication they cannot replace face-to-face communication in terms of impact and effectiveness. Indeed, the caution required when using technical communication channels can be problematic, as is further explained in Chapter Ten.

WHAT IS ONE-TO-ONE COMMUNICATION?

Before giving practical advice on how to be effective in one-to-one communication, a few basic definitions will be helpful. Decker (1997), for example, defined this type of communication as comprising nine behavioural skills.

1. Eye communication
2. Posture and movement
3. Gestures and facial expression
4. Dress and appearance
5. Voice and voice variety
6. Language, pauses and non-words
7. Listener involvement
8. Using humour
9. The natural self

He describes non-words as 'um's', 'er's' and 'ah's'. The idea of the natural self centres on understanding your natural strengths and building weaknesses into strengths. Another definition by Hargie (1997) considers core communication skills as consisting of:

- Non-verbal behaviour
- Questioning
- Reinforcement
- Reflecting
- Explaining
- Self-disclosure
- The process of listening
- Humour and laughter

This chapter will consider some of these elements in more detail later. Many will come as no surprise, yet the opportunity to focus on them will, it is hoped, provide useful insight.

One-to-one communication

THE CLINICAL PROFESSIONAL AS COMMUNICATOR

One of the most important skills for clinical or nurse managers is a well-developed capability as a communicator. Clinical professionals communicate with or talk to many people every day of the working week. They talk to other clinical staff at all levels in the hierarchy. They talk to patients and relatives. They talk with other professionals: doctors from every level, occupational therapists, physiotherapists, dieticians, social workers, health visitors, midwives and other health care professionals. They talk with administrative staff, domiciliary staff and catering staff. The list is never ending.

From the moment many non-clinical managers set off to work they probably think about how they will be communicating with others for that day. They will have decided what to wear, particularly if an important meeting is to take place. Image and presentation are critical in one-to-one communication as first impressions commonly set the tone in meetings. Image alone communicates something to others. We all make assumptions and have attitudes about others and this is usually based on our first impression of the person.

How you look matters. There are those who insist that it does not matter what you wear to work. They might assert that if a person dresses too smartly or 'power dresses', this creates barriers. Many clinical professionals, for example, do not wear uniform to work, preferring an informal style of dress. What does this communicate? What image are they portraying of the service or organisation they represent? What do the patients think? Some will say it is what you do at work that matters and it would be foolish to disagree with this point of view. However, your appearance will communicate something about you before you open your mouth. In this instance casual dress and appearance may not be acceptable to others and this needs to be borne in mind if this prevails in your clinical area. Dressing more formally for an important meeting outside the unit, for example, might have a positive influence on success.

WORKING RELATIONSHIPS

One of the factors affecting communication with others is your working relationship with them. As a clinical manager you will have many and varied working relationships with colleagues. In some of these relationships you will hold power and authority, especially if you act as a line manager. This will affect how colleagues communicate with you. Before you have even started to talk with them other dynamics will be at play. What does the member of staff want from you? What do you want from them? Sometimes, without you knowing why, because you are a manager, you can be perceived negatively by that person. They may have had negative experiences with other managers or people in authority and you become for them another 'withholder' or potentially difficult encounter. In such situations communication is already difficult before you start. You may become involved in a power struggle with someone. You may be with someone who thinks they could do your job better than you. All these factors can cause problems and the skilled manager needs to be aware of this and devise approaches to ameliorate it and reduce the stress such situations can cause.

STRESS LEVELS AND COMMUNICATION

How do you communicate when you are feeling stressed? Feeling stressed affects the way we relate to others. We are more irritable, short tempered and prone to making irrational decisions. Does this come across to others? As a clinical manager it goes without saying that you have a very stressful job. You are sometimes 'piggy in the middle'. There are demands being made on you from above by management and from below by your colleagues, patients or clients. Somehow clinical professionals have to juggle all these demands, balance them and communicate a response that satisfies all parties. This is not easy, particularly when stress levels are high.

THE ROLE OF THE SENSES IN ONE-TO-ONE COMMUNICATION

Take some time to consider how you communicate. What are the senses that you use? Who do you communicate with? Why do you communicate with others? What is the importance of communication in your role as a clinical manager?

The sense of hearing allows people to talk to each other and in the case of telephone calls, is the only one used to get the message across. Because of this single sense communication it is one of the simplest methods to use but, like many simple things, has potential drawbacks. The quality of information in a telephone message can be compromised by the lack of reinforcement from messages using other senses.

Sight is for most people the dominant sense. In face-to-face communications people reinforce messages sent using sound with the use of gestures, facial expression and more subtle body language.

Touch is used in more intimate messages. Most forms of touch have social taboos applying to their use. Hitting and pushing are discouraged from an early age. In a work context managers who are too free with their personal contact lay themselves open to allegations of overfamiliarity from their staff.

The sense catalogue is completed by taste and smell. There are practical limits to the use of these senses but it is worth remembering how they can interfere with good communication. If I serve a cup of dark, bitter coffee to someone when I am attempting to find out information from them it can be distracting to the point where it prevents the free exchange of information. The person might feel that they need to curtail the conversation so that they can go and wash their mouth out. They will also be less likely to put themselves in a similar position again which will reduce the opportunity for communication in the future.

MODELS OF COMMUNICATION

It is important to bear in mind when considering any sort of model that it is a schematic representation of, in this case, how communication occurs and what elements are thought to be involved. It is not an accurate representation of real life. Models therefore can usefully guide our thinking and understanding but cannot always be applied directly in real situations.

The communication model outlined in Figure 2.1 is very simple. A practical example of this type of one-to-one communication might be you reading this book. The author of this chapter is the sender of the message and the message is represented by the words printed on the page. You as the reader are the recipient. If this is taken a step further and there was a need to set up a one-to-one verbal communication the model would become more complex. This is set out in schematic form in Figure 2.2.

Feedback allows the sender to alter or embellish the message to increase the chances of the meaning being understood by the recipient or for subtle changes in the message to be made. It can be in the form of verbal and non-verbal cues and is considered

Personal communication

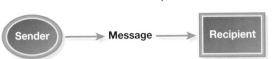

Figure 2.1 A simple model of communication.

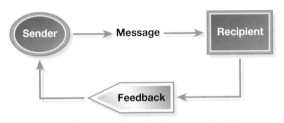

Figure 2.2 A simple model of verbal communication.

in this model to be necessary to keep the communication developing.

Consider ways that feedback is denied by a recipient and the results of that tactic. Someone who asks a passer-by for some spare change, for example, tries to make eye contact with the person. If eye contact is achieved there is a very good chance of a donation. If eye contact is not achieved because the person targeted avoids it then it is probable that no money will be forthcoming. The listener can make a conscious choice to prevent the communication by refusing to acknowledge that the message has been received. A similar example in the health care setting might be a situation wherein you as a manager have to deal with a difficult situation with a colleague who avoids eye contact during a discussion as they do not wish to admit guilt or be admonished.

The next stage of complexity for one-to-one communication is illustrated in Figure 2.3. Nearly all communication is two-way and this model advocated by Schramm (1965) could be reversed each time the speaker changes within the conversation. Schramm does not see feedback as an explicit part of his model. The person who initiates the message (encoder) needs to be aware that a message is required. They need to be aware of a 'communications gap' and the need to encode their message in such a way as to promote

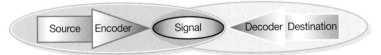

Figure 2.3 A more complex model of communication (adapted from Schramm 1965).

One-to-one communication

understanding on the part of the listener or receiver (decoder). As will be shown later, this involves more than getting the words right.

The personality of the sender will also influence willingness to communicate. Introverted people tend to avoid communicating, as do people who are depressed. Some of us use every opportunity, valid or not, to communicate with others. People make judgements about how friendly, unfriendly, helpful or unhelpful others are. This provides immediate feedback through the subtle use of body language and as long as the sender is receptive to the message being sent, the chances of successfully sending the message are improved.

The objectives of the sender need to be clear before communication starts; planning communication is one of the most powerful strategies for developing its effectiveness. It can be seen as being like a lever. Implementing communication without planning will undoubtedly create an effect, though this may not be the desired one. However, planning gives the implementation greater leverage by enabling a degree of certainty about the result and some contingency in situations where things do not go according to plan. Consequently it helps to try to plan how you intend to get your meaning across. This can be achieved by gaining prior knowledge of the person you intend to communicate with and their potential reaction to what you have to say. In addition, you may need to think about what you want the outcomes to be. Naturally this does not work in all situations, especially when communicating in a situation for which you have not prepared. This emphasises the need always to be aware of verbal and non-verbal cues to assist in maximising your effectiveness in communication.

COMPOSITION OF A MESSAGE

The way in which a message is composed or constructed has an effect on the result of that communication. Consider the language that is used to communicate. This chapter is written in English rather than any other language for the obvious reason that the potential audience is going to understand the message best in that language. American English could have been used with almost the same effect although some readers might object and crucially some key words might not be the same or others might be used in critically different ways.

In our professional lives particular interest groups use particular sets of words. Nurses talking to other nurses use a language that contains words and abbreviations learnt through common experience and teaching. Physiotherapists, doctors and other professionals do the same. Their 'languages' are sufficiently different from others to lead, at times, to failures in understanding. As a clinical manager, you may find talking to a finance manager difficult. They will use a lot of accounting terms not, you hope, to confuse you but to convey what they mean. This said, it is up to the sender to encode the message in ways that will be readily understood by the recipient. This is the basis for intelligible and effective interpersonal or one-to-one communication. The message consists not only of the words but also voice and body language.

As has been previously stated the sender needs to understand that there is a need to communicate. They need to have an understanding of the needs of others as well as an effective appreciation of the perspective of others. This can be seen as building on the strengths of communication with patients that clinical staff utilise in their everyday work so that it can be understood or appreciated in a managerial context.

ELEMENTS OF A MESSAGE

The message itself is the only part of communication that is common to the sender and the recipient. Argyle (1970) identified the elements of a message as consisting of body language, voice tonality and words and saw the impact of each of these elements as not being proportionate to one another. Figure 2.4 indicates the relative importance of each element.

According to this diagram, in communicating with others, body language has the most impact on the message being conveyed.

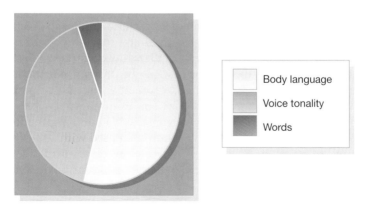

Body language
Voice tonality
Words

Figure 2.4 Elements of a message (Argyle 1970, with permission from Routledge).

What people say is deemed to be of least importance. This is particularly important to consider when speaking to professionals from other disciplines. Body language, for example, may confirm or deny preexisting perceptions one group has about another which is why body language and appearance are so important in communication between clinicians and non-clinical managers. The words used to communicate will convey the necessary details, but this may not be fully appreciated if the mind of the recipient is focused on body language which may be conveying a negative or contrary message.

Behavioural skills

If we refer back to the behavioural skills identified by Decker (p. 27) at least six of the nine skills can be deemed as either directly related to body language or as having a crucial influence on it: eye communication, posture and movement, gestures and facial movement, dress and appearance, listener involvement and the natural self (i.e. self-confidence). These can be considered from a practical point of view under the following headings.

Eyes

The face tends to be the part of a person that others focus on first. Eyes are the most important indicator and are the first thing that a person will look at. How, for example, do you make eye contact with someone? Do you look at them directly, indirectly or not at all? Many feelings can be expressed with the eyes ranging from happiness through sadness and disappointment to anger. We all know what it is like to be on the receiving end of an angry stare. Facial expressions say more than anything else. It pays to give this aspect of communication some thought and to even go into non-critical conversations, for example, with the aim of noting how eye contact is made and the lessons that can be drawn from this. Are people put off by a direct stare? Does averting the eyes lead the other person to become anxious? This exercise will enable you to become comfortable with eye contact while adopting the most effective approach in different situations.

The body

As Argyle (1970) states, the body often sends messages more strongly than words. A slouch indicates disinterest. An upright posture indicates formality. The way we sit or stand can say a lot suggesting whether one is tense or relaxed. Crossing your arms in front of your body can indicate a defensive posture. Constant bodily movement signals anxiety. Do you lean forward when talking or sit back? What does such a posture say about you? Leaning forward can indicate interest and leaning backwards can indicate lack of interest.

Where one chooses to sit or stand in relation to someone else is important. Sitting side by side makes it harder to achieve eye contact. Having one's personal space invaded by someone standing or sitting too closely is uncomfortable and can be perceived as threatening. Being touched, especially if this is deemed to be inappropriate, can be off-putting, especially if you don't know an individual well.

Hands and arms are used by different cultures to a greater or lesser extent. Many cultural or ethnic groups also place greater emphasis on the importance of contact or touch. It is harder to concentrate on what someone is saying if they are waving their arms around as you tend to focus on the movement. This said, awareness of cultural or ethnic differences can make a critical difference to the success of communication. It is important, therefore, to take account of this, especially as the government rightly celebrates and encourages diversity in the NHS and public sector.

Dress

The way people dress provides clues as to their role and status and the importance they attribute to the situation they are in. An interview candidate with scruffy clothes is sending a clear message about their attitude to the interview. There was a trend in the 1980s and early 1990s to 'power dress'. The idea was to impress people with clothes that looked business-like, decisive and smart in the expectation that this would be seen as a reflection of the wearer's character also. The key is, as stated before, to plan ahead. It may not be appropriate, relevant or practical to wear a suit in all situations but consideration of neatness in personal appearance will significantly improve the chances of success and may even avoid undue stereotyping.

Many people, notably in management positions in America, even go so far as to consult colour analysts to advise on the best colours for them. Such advice even covered the colours to use in key scenarios. While this may be deemed excessive in Britain, it does indicate how perceptions of an individual are built on more than words in one-to-one situations.

One-to-one communication

Vocal tone

The tone of your voice is obviously important in trying to get a message across. The pace of your words is also important. Do you speak too quickly or slowly? Is your voice highpitched or low? Does your voice change if you are anxious? Are you loud or quiet? The following aspects of a situation can be indicated by tone.

● Feelings – love, hate, happiness, sadness, boredom, excitement, interest
● Position – superiority, inferiority, comradeship
● Relationship – friendly, business-like, teaching, preaching, antagonistic, loving

Voice pitch (that is, whether the voice is shrill, deep or perceived as mid range) can convey a range of things, including gender, age, status, social class, fear and anxiety, among others. If a problem is identified in this area coaching can be useful in providing a remedy if tone blocks a person's ability to communicate effectively. Indeed, if a problem becomes apparent it is often best to ask a person you trust and whose opinion will be accurate before acting to change tonal problems.

Speed

Speed of delivery of speech in one-to-one situations is important. Speech that is too fast can confuse or intimidate the listener, especially if the discussion contains new or technical terminology. It is important therefore to speak slowly enough to be understood but not too slowly to bore.

It is useful to train yourself to use silence or pauses to allow the listener to assimilate what you have said. This also emphasises the importance of effective listening and spotting cues on the part of the listener when you are speaking.

Words

Lastly, the words you use are necessary for accuracy and meaning, in spite of the academic view that they are the least important part of the message. Words are important but should not detract from or block other elements of the message. People developing their communications skills tend to concentrate on the words to the exclusion of voice and body. The key issue here is that while different weights are attached to the elements of a message, each is impor-

Personal communication

tant in its own right. The work of Argyle (1970), for example, is important in drawing our attention to what constitutes an effective message. As with all models, it should guide our thinking so that we can, as our experience grows, use this knowledge to perfect our communication skills.

LISTENING

McKay et al (1993) differentiate between real and pseudo-listening. They say 'real listening' is based on the intention to do one of four things:

1. understand someone
2. enjoy someone
3. learn something
4. give help or solace.

They go further to say that 'pseudo-listening' is intended to meet the listener's own needs by:

- making people think you're interested so they will like you
- being alert to see if you are in danger of getting rejected
- listening for one specific piece of information and ignoring everything else
- buying time to prepare your next comment
- half-listening so that someone will listen to you
- listening to find someone's vulnerabilities or to take advantage
- looking for the weak points in an argument so you can always be right, listening to get ammunition for attack
- checking to see how people are reacting, making sure you produce the desired effect
- half-listening because a good, kind or nice person would
- half-listening because you don't know how to get away without hurting or offending someone.

This would suggest that listening is rather more than simply 'hearing 'what is being said. This leads on to an awareness of active listening, a term which has become popular in the health care sector in recent years. Active listening is a skill mentioned by many writers on interpersonal communications. There are, broadly, four elements to it:

- clarifying (including paraphrasing)
- drawing out
- suspending judgement
- physical attending and giving feedback.

One-to-one communication

Clarifying is a process of checking that what you have understood is the same as the meaning that the speaker transmitted. One way of doing this would be to question the speaker about their meaning. A softer and more enabling approach would be to paraphrase what you had just heard using sentences starting with 'What I hear you saying is . . .' or 'In other words . . . ' or 'So basically how you felt was . . . ', followed by your interpretation of what the speaker had just said in your own words.

Drawing out is another useful way of getting more information to increase your chances of getting the right message. Ask 'open' questions which cannot be answered with just 'yes' or 'no'. Try questions starting with 'What . . . ?' or 'How do you know . . . ?' or if the speaker is working with 'facts', ask them about 'feelings' and vice versa. Use questions like 'How do you feel about . . . ?' or 'How can that be substantiated?'.

Suspending judgement is one of the hardest active listening skills to practise. It requires the listener to put aside their prejudices and preconceptions. To suspend judgement, try to listen positively. Do not reject others' ideas until you have heard them fully, asked questions and considered the replies. Give responses that allow the other person to argue their case to the full and put up reasoned counter-arguments that acknowledge an individual's right to express their opinions and ideas without ridicule.

Attentiveness and giving feedback are required to encourage a speaker to express themselves clearly and fully. To encourage people to continue talking, use nods of the head. Encouraging speakers who use too many 'um's and 'ah's to be more precise in what they say is important while giving them proper time to express themselves. Maintain good eye contact, keep an open posture and mirror their non-verbal signals.

At this stage it might be worth considering what behaviour in others makes it difficult for you to communicate with them. How do you feel if a person listening to you does one or more of the following?

- Folds their arms and raises their shoulders
- Stares straight in your eyes for prolonged periods
- Frowns
- Gets very close to you, particularly when you are seated and they are standing
- Does not look at you
- Looks at the floor
- Doodles
- Yawns

- Checks the time
- Keeps looking around

It is highly likely that you would react negatively to such behaviour. This is why it is so important to minimise such actions on your own part when communicating face to face.

CONCLUSION

This chapter has attempted to consider the often complex business of one-to-one communication in terms of its basic elements. This is not to belittle the importance of such communication but to provide a practical means of understanding how we communicate in this way, what is involved and how we can make a start to improve the way we relate directly to other people in communicating our thoughts, ideas or intentions. A couple of quotes from Herda & Messerschmidt (1991) sum things up very well.

> A manager skilled in communication is one who knows how to listen and can utilise the power of language as a resource to bring employees to their full creative capacities, resulting in useful and appropriate actions.

> A competent speaker needs only to use language that is comprehended but a communicator needs to be oriented towards reaching mutual understanding.

Consider all elements of communication and it should be possible to improve how we as health care professionals communicate. This set of skills will be required more and more as the health care setting becomes more complex and the requirement grows to explain to others what we do in order to advance our work.

Practice checklist

Always consider how non-verbal behaviour or body language impacts on one-to-one communication.

- Consider the appropriateness of dress and/or appearance prior to meetings or entering into one-to-one discussions.
- Reflect on working relationships and how these affect communication, particularly at an interpersonal level.
- Always take evidence of stress into account when assessing reactions to episodes of one-to-one communication.
- Think of the role of the senses in communciation, particularly taking into account the importance of eye contact, the use of touch (if appropriate) and hearing.

One-to-one communication

Practice checklist (*Cont.*)

- Remember, the tone of voice influences reactions to inter-personal communications.
- Try to remember that one-to-one communication, in simple terms an encoded message being sent to a recipient, places particular emphasis on the need to be aware of the perspective and perception of the recipient to ensure that the correct message is conveyed.
- It is important not to speak too quickly and to ensure that language used is understood by the recipient.
- Always listen carefully to responses and indicate the appropriate level of engagement in responses to what is being said.
- Be careful to monitor and check feedback during one-to-one communication, as this provides vital information on how the recipient is reacting to what is being said and how the sender can alter their approach as a means of ensuring a more positive outcome.

Discussion questions

- What examples can you recall of situations where one-to-one communication led to a negative or poor outcome?
- What examples can you recall of situations where one-to-one communication led to a positive outcome?
- Do you feel that appearance and dress, as stated in the preceding chapter, impact on the effectiveness of one-to-one communication in today's National Health Service?
- Does the use of body language, voice tone, eye contact and listening skills vary from one professional group to another (in your opinion)?
- Do you believe that different aspects of one-to-one communication, as discussed in the preceding chapter, impact on the way in which clinical professionals talk to other clinical professionals and clinical professionals talk to non-clinical professionals?

References

Argyle M 1970 Bodily communication, 2nd edn. Routledge, London
Decker B 1997 How to communicate effectively. Kogan Page, London
Hargie ODW (ed) 1997 The handbook of communication skills. Routledge, London

Personal communication

Herda E, Messerschmidt DA 1991 From words to actions. Leadership and Organisation Development Journal 12(1): 24–25

Lloyd P 1994 Hard news. Health Service Journal 2 June: 18–20

McKay M, Davis M, Fanning P 1993 Messages: the communication book. New Harbinger Publications, Oakland, California

Schramm W 1965 The process and effects of mass communication. University of Illinois Press, Champaign, Illinois

Further reading

Clark RA 1984 Persuasive messages. Harper and Row, New York

Gouran D, Wiethoff WE, Doelger JA 1994 Mastering communication, 2nd edn. Allyn and Bacon, Boston

Griffin EM 1997 A first look at communication theory, 3rd edn. McGraw-Hill, New York

Hough A 1987 Communication in health care. Physiotherapy 73(2): 56–59

Hybels S, Weaver RL 1989 Communicating effectively, 5th edn. McGraw-Hill, Boston

Knapp M 1984 Interpersonal communication and human relationships. Allyn and Bacon, Boston

Kurtz S, Silverman J, Draper J 1998 Teaching and learning communication skill in medicine. Radcliffe Medical Press, Abingdon

Lloyd M, Bor R 1996 Basic communication skills. In: Communication skills for medicine. Churchill Livingstone, London

Miller C 1994 The empowered communicator. Broadman and Holman, Nashville, Tennessee

Noonan P 1998 Simply speaking. Regan Books, New York

Scott MD, Brydon SR 1997 Dimensions of communication: an introduction. Mayfield, Mountain View, California

Trenholm S 1995 Thinking through communication: an introduction to the study of human communication. Allyn and Bacon, Boston

Zueschner R 1997 Communicating today. Allyn and Bacon, Boston

One-to-one communication

Application **2:1**
Mark Darley

Appearance: a personal development plan

As has been stated in the main chapter, appearance is a key element of communication. What follows is an outline for analysing this aspect of your approach to work as a means of determining improvements, should this be deemed necessary. In each instance, an outline personal development plan is provided to help you explore these issues.

ASSESSMENT

First, examine your appearance by using some or all of the following:

- mirror
- video camera with audio switched off
- other people (manager, peers, subordinates, partner).

Audit your appearance as if you were seeing yourself for the first time. What overall impression do you make? Consider height, weight, grooming, dress (style, quality, upkeep), stance and facial expression.

Personal development plan: appearance

I will concentrate on changing: By this date

1 . . . . / . . . . / . . . .
2 . . . . / . . . . / . . . .
3 . . . . / . . . . / . . . .

I will know I have succeeded when:

1 . . . .
2 . . . .
3 . . . .

For each item you should set a measurable improvement and a target date for the change. Remember that behavioural change is often difficult to achieve quickly. Habits reinforced over a lifetime do not lend themselves to instant modification and practice will be needed.

Listen to your voice by using some or all of the following:

- tape recorder
- video camera with audio switched on
- other people (manager, peers, subordinates, partner).

Audit your voice as if you were hearing yourself for the first time. What is the overall impression? Think about volume, pitch, tone, persistence, intonation, clarity, accent and speed.

Personal development plan: voice

I will concentrate on changing:	By this date
1	...../...../....
2	...../...../....
3	...../...../....

I will know I have succeeded when:

1 ....
2 ....
3 ....

Look at your body language by using some or all of the following:

- mirror
- video camera with audio switched off
- other people.

Audit your body language as if you were seeing yourself for the first time. What is the overall impression? Consider stance, eye contact, smiles, frowns, mouth movements, hand and arm movements, head movements, whole-body movements, hand movements.

Personal development plan: body language

I will concentrate on changing:	By this date
1	...../...../....
2	...../...../....
3	...../...../....

I will know I have succeeded when:

1 ....
2 ....
3 ....

Appearance: a personal development plan

ACTION

Once you have decided which things you wish to change, take the nine items from the above lists and place them in priority order. Consider what the consequences would be of changing, what the consequences would be of not changing and how much effort will be required to achieve change.

Now consider which six of the nine items you could best learn to live with and leave them for later. Take the three items you really want to work on and consider these for a detailed development plan. Ask yourself the following questions.

- Why do I do this thing?
- Does it have any practical purpose?
- What would happen if I stopped or changed it?
- Would I do something different that I would like even less?

You will need to monitor your progress towards your goals. A powerful way of doing this is to use a reflective diary. At the end of each day spend a few minutes recording the way in which you handled communications in the last 24 hours. It needn't take very long as you can do this in note form – it is for your use only.

VOICE

Record yourself on tape. If you are using a video camera to do this do not look at the image but concentrate on the voice alone. What do you like about the sound of your own voice? What do you want to change? Check this out with other people to see if they hear you in the same way as you hear yourself. Use your recording to do this so that both of you are listening to the same example of your voice. Think about your voice in terms of pitch. Try out on tape talking in a high pitch, a normal pitch and a low pitch. Are there times when you unconsciously change the pitch? When you are under stress, does the pitch tend to become higher? When you feel fully in control does the pitch tend to lower? If you are aware of these changes then you can start to develop a voice that you want others to hear. Behavioural characteristics such as voice pitch have been learnt over a lifetime so it is unlikely that you will be able to change them totally overnight.

Volume of voice is more difficult to assess on tape. If you are a quiet speaker you are no doubt aware of this already. People ask you to repeat things. Perhaps they do not hear you at all, particularly in crowded or noisy environments. Sometimes they give more obvious signs such as cupping their hands behind their ears to try to improve their listening ability. Try out your voice while sitting and while standing. Experiment with taking one or two deep breaths before speaking and consciously dropping your shoulders and relaxing your diaphragm muscles. The more air you have in your lungs, the easier it will be to make a big noise! Choose a safe environment (perhaps when you are driving in your car alone but do not be distracted from the driving) and try shouting as loud as you can. Remember what it is that you do with your body to increase the volume of your voice.

Test it out by involving a colleague in an experiment. Tell them that you want to try out your communication skills by getting them to listen to something you have to say. Explain that you are trying to assess your performance as a communicator but do not tell them how you are going to measure it. Have a prepared script that lasts for 2–3 minutes together with a list of important points that you want to get over. After reading the script to the other person in an environment conducive to good communication (quiet, interruption free, comfortable), ask them to recall what you have told them. Mark off the points that the listener recalls accurately. Thank the person for their assistance and explain again that the exercise was to give you feedback on your ability to communicate and not to test their powers of recall.

Appearance: a personal development plan

Application **2:2**

Mark Darley

Listening skills exercise

With another two like-minded people, try the following exercise. It is also possible to do this with one other person and a video camera.

Decide on a topic each of you will talk on for 2 minutes. Spend 10 minutes planning out what you are going to say on your own. One person then talks to another person while the third person (or the video camera) observes the interaction. After 2 minutes swap roles so that each person talks and each person listens.

What the person is talking about is unimportant. The listener should use active listening skills (clarifying, drawing out, suspending judgement and physical attending). The observer should be prepared to feed back performance of active listening skills.

After each interaction, 10 minutes should be spent on feedback. First the speaker should tell the listener how they perceived the listener's active listening skills. Second, the observer should give feedback or the video playback should be watched and critiqued. The exercise should be repeated for each participant.

The final stage of this exercise is to devise an action plan for each individual by considering the following.

Box 2.2.1

My active listening skills strengths are:

1 . . . .

2 . . . .

3 . . . .

My active listening skills weaknesses are:

1 . . . .

2 . . . .

3 . . . .

I will build on my strengths by:

1 . . . .

2 . . . .

3 . . . .

I will strengthen my weaknesses by:

1 . . . .

2 . . . .

3 . . . .

If you have found things that are important to work on, it may be worth considering setting targets for change and measuring the outcomes.

Some bad habits when listening

- Advising
- Being irrelevant
- Blaming
- Diagnosing
- Directing and leading
- Distracting
- Faking attention
- Getting angry
- Humouring
- Ignoring the other's feelings
- Inappropriately talking about yourself
- Interrogating
- Judging and evaluating
- Labelling
- Moralising
- Overinterpreting
- Putting time constraints on the other person
- Reassuring
- Teaching

How many of the above can you see in others? How many can you see in yourself?

Chapter **Three**

Influencing and negotiating skills

Anne Palmer

Personal communication

OVERVIEW

In this chapter the author provides a detailed insight into the mechanics of negotiation and how clinical professionals (mostly nurses in this case) can use these skills.

As with so many of the key skills and techniques related to communication in the modern health care industry, the ability to negotiate is becoming ever more important to clinical professionals. Whether it is attending a key meeting to negotiate for resources or involvement in a human resource matter, the ability to negotiate effectively will at the very least put you on an equal footing with non-clinical managers who are possibly more used to using such skills. Anne Palmer has provided an excellent overview of key points to guide interested practitioners in developing their skills and understanding the context in which to use them.

INTRODUCTION

Influencing and persuading are essential management skills which lie at the very heart of effective negotiation (Fowler 1996). They are also necessary skills for building effective relationships and improving communication in management (Cleeton & Sharman 2000). Those experienced in negotiation techniques have suggested that we live in an age of negotiating where all aspects of our lives are subject to some degree of negotiation (Kennedy et al 1987).

While negotiation can be considered a complex process it is interesting to note that we use the same negotiation skills whether we are:

- buying a house
- in dispute with neighbours
- collaborating with individuals or groups.

If we accept that nearly all informal daily activity involves some use of negotiation skills, then it appears reasonable to suggest that these are necessary skills for those working together and those who have to manage others. Being able to negotiate well is particularly important for nurse managers who at some juncture will make attempts at influencing and persuading others to meet the challenges and current demands of providing quality health care. Such influencing and persuading skills will be evident in encouraging others to:

- take on new activities, roles and responsibilities
- make changes to their practice
- perform well in a demoralised service
- work together more effectively.

The focus for this chapter concerns the process of negotiation, what it is and how to be successful in achieving what you want when negotiating. It also concerns the influencing, persuading and bargaining skills that form part of any negotiation so that you, the manager, can play an active part in influencing and changing practice. This has added importance particularly now that working collaboratively has become a key aspect of current NHS policy and greater emphasis is being placed on the need for collaboration in the health service (DoH 2000). This adds to the challenge of the manager's working environment, where the emphasis is on ensuring an evidence-based culture and pressing quality imperatives. Such challenges are making their demands felt and managers have an increasing need to develop their powers of persuasion.

Negotiating is therefore an important aspect of the nurse or clinical manager's portfolio of personal and professional competencies. If this is not already evident it will become increasingly so as clinical managers seek to manage and deliver a service within an organisational climate where there are staff and skill shortages and

Influencing and negotiating skills

where morale may be low (Tovey 2000). There is also growing emphasis on collaborative working and initiatives to ensure that professions and disciplines work and learn together (Barr 1996, Carpenter 1995). Poor collaboration results in mistakes, resource wastage and professionals taking on too much (Barr 2001). As a result patients or service users may become alienated and their needs may be ignored.

Developing effective communication skills, starting with the interpersonal aspects that encourage clear communication and a critical dialogue between others, is a central feature of negotiation. These skills can help health care professionals to negotiate within their organisations and, increasingly, across the intersector or interagency boundaries to effect a seamless service. Other occupational groups are also recognising the need to consider effective communication and negotiation skills, as demonstrated by the police. Recent poor publicity and criticism of police working have led to a concerted drive for partnership with other public sector workers (Metropolitan Police Service 2000).

This chapter offers a framework in which the skills and behaviours involved in successful negotiations can be explored and reflected upon. The proposed framework involves the phases of preparation, orchestration and evaluation, which are considered as the key aspects necessary for negotiation in practice (Fig. 3.1). Preparation concerns setting the scene for the negotiations, while orchestration relates to the considerations that are important in presenting your case. The third aspect, evaluation, revolves around

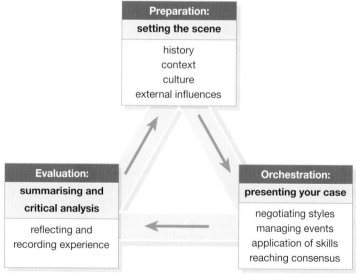

Figure 3.1 A negotiation framework.

the reflecting and recording issues that are essential in determining what occurred and what you learnt. These are considered the necessary phases in helping you become a successful negotiator and someone adept at influencing and changing practice. First, however, we need to consider what negotiation is and what it involves.

DEFINING NEGOTIATION

In formal management terms negotiation is a situation where two or more individuals have to reach an agreement in order to change something or make progress. It is an activity that seeks to reach agreement between two or more different starting positions (Honey 1988). In less formal language, it involves bargaining which means making a deal, getting agreement and seeing the deal implemented. It can be 'viewed as a constructive process that contributes to an organisation's success, not as a battle of preservation of personal or corporate power or prestige' (Fowler 1996, p. viii). Successful negotiation also involves influencing another's views or beliefs and persuading them to change or getting them to come around to your point of view. This process of persuasion involves exploring what may initially appear as diverse views or perspectives, hearing all sides of the argument and reaching some form of agreement or consensus (Fowler 1996, Wolfe 1990).

In an ideal world, when negotiating, you would get everything you wanted, agree to everything the other individual or parties wanted, meet everyone's expectations and all participants would be contented. All types of negotiation, be they informal or formal, have one significant factor in common: the parties (or individuals) involved have varying degrees of power but not absolute power over each other. It is this factor that makes the art of influencing and persuading and the skill of negotiating a complex and highly engaging process. Weightman (1996) contends that influencing others to work towards making decisions or behaving in a manner that they may not have considered is central to working within organisations. She offers three models of behaviour in influencing others at work. These are the psychoanalysis, behaviourism and humanistic psychology models.

Weightman's analysis suggests that in attempting to influence others, you should consider yourself, the other person/parties involved, the interaction about to occur and the environment in which this will take place. These are essential considerations forming part of the negotiating process that is explored in the discussions that follow. Those wishing to explore issues around such

Influencing and negotiating skills

51

models should refer to texts that add to our understanding of human relations and interactions at work (Clampitt 1991, Obholzer & Roberts 1994, Pennington 2001).

An effective way of visualising the negotiation process in nursing is to consider Peplau's model of nursing (Peplau 1952). Although this was published many years ago the ideas and deliberations still have resonance today. They help us appreciate the process of negotiation in action, at an individual patient, service user and practitioner level. In Peplau's view the nurse and the patient or user may start from completely different perspectives concerning the individual needs and responses to treatment or care. Each party has to negotiate through social interaction to reach agreement on the aims and outcomes of treatment and care required. The nurse is required to appreciate the patient's or user's perspective identified from the history, social interactions and an understanding of the diagnosis. The two parties have to reach agreement and this involves applying the skills of communication and negotiation.

Such a negotiating process commonly involves a verbal interaction between those involved that requires the application of the range of social interactions and communicative skills explored in the other chapters of this book. In talking and discussing care, the salient points can be shared but it is when negotiation is introduced to the interaction that common concerns and uncovering of each other's expectations can be more easily explored. Negotiation in this situation promotes an atmosphere of give and take where trust and respect can develop as the issues are aired and both parties, the nurse and patient or user, can agree on how to proceed.

Negotiation is a complex process influenced by a range of factors that have to be considered and thought through, if the process is to be a success. Often such factors are outside your jurisdiction or control and it is this that makes negotiating an exciting prospect for creative and astute managers willing to take risks. In appreciating and understanding negotiation it is also important to consider the language that may be used during the process.

THE LANGUAGE OF NEGOTIATION

Negotiation is a complex process because each person negotiating believes that by discussing the salient issues and putting their argument (the negotiation), they will persuade the other person to modify their original position and come round to their point of view. This situation relies on each person's ability to engage in a

Personal communication

meaningful dialogue and a willingness to compromise (work towards a settlement). It also involves conciliation and concessions to reach a consensus and these terms are explained in Box 3.1.

It is important to note that negotiation is not coercion, as it is not forcing someone to come over to your position and it is not using power and authority over another to make them take on your perspective. It involves two or more negotiating partners who need each other's, or believe they need each other's, involvement and commitment in achieving an agreed outcome or consensus. By the same token, it is obvious that common interests do draw individuals or groups together to negotiate and help them to maintain contact through the process. These common interests may be related to the need to change, in implementing policy or in responding to a problem at work (see Case study 3.1).

Box 3.1 Common terms used in negotiation

Conciliation This is the agreement to a condition put forward by the other side (your negotiating partner) to make them more agreeable to the negotiation process. It often means giving up something you considered important. This is an important part of the negotiation as it can speed up the process or restart discussions if the process has faltered.

Concession Agreement to a condition that you did not initially want. It usually means that you do not get any equivalent or compensating agreement from your negotiating partner.

Compromise This is the trading of concessions so that neither of you gets everything you originally wanted but both sides are satisfied by the outcome.

Consensus This occurs when you and your negotiating partner agree to an issue or outcome.

Case study 3.1 Negotiating for a better transport system

These issues are evident in the negotiations under way in the attempt to develop the London Tube network. The common interests shared by the government, the management of London Transport and representatives of the various unions relate to maintaining the service. Current negotiations involve how to develop an ageing transport system at a time when resources are restricted and passenger concerns growing. Common issues draw the various factions to the negotiating arena; however, how they achieve the aims of implementing an agreed strategy will form the basis for the negotiations. The factors influencing the negotiations are those

Influencing and negotiating skills

Personal communication

Case study 3.1 (*Cont.*)

commonly identified in any negotiation process but primarily relate, in this author's view, to the nature of the relationships of the parties involved.

It is important to remember when considering the factors that affect negotiations that each negotiator will have some degree of influence or power (real or assumed) over another's ability to act. In the case of London Transport, the management employs the workers and has the power to sack them, while the workers deliver the service and have the power to strike and cause disruption. At the same time, the government has the power to press home new policies that require the application of private funding to complement what is essentially a public service. The government's power lies in the ability to withdraw funding from a public utility.

Discussion

The issues emerging here are that individuals and parties have to perceive some benefits in negotiating together and that there should be perceptions that there is an equal balance of power. This influences those involved and brings the negotiating sides together to reach a consensus and work at gaining compliance to take any initiatives forward. If there is an imbalance and one individual or party is too powerful, with the other powerless, there is limited scope for negotiation and if outcomes are forced through this may lead to disruptions and resistance to change. This was evident in the NHS in the early 1970s when a culture of strong unions and demanding professional bodies in negotiation with management led to disruptions to the service. This resulted in a culture in which the politics of conflict and disillusionment were evident (Klein 1989).

Negotiating skills do not give managers power in situations where they did not have it previously but they do allow the power that exists to be used more effectively. This makes negotiating an interesting prospect for nurse managers in public and private health sectors, at a time when resources are increasingly being rationed and professional uncertainty exists. There may also be insecurities about roles and an increasing focus on short-term responsibilities and outcomes (Meads & Ashcroft 2000). Negotiation may appear as a daunting prospect as nurse managers in particular have to enter into discussions or negotiations with other disciplines or professions that have traditionally viewed themselves as superior or are unwilling to challenge their stereotypes of the nurse's role and responsibilities (Davies 1995,

Wicks 1998). This is evident in Case study 3.2 where there is an unequal distribution of power during negotiations with inappropriate perceptions of one group's roles and responsibilities.

Case study 3.2   Power and non-negotiation

The decision to reduce junior doctors' hours was taken following consultation and the publication of the report *The New Deal* (DoH 1991), which identified the pressures on junior doctors. Initial negotiations for implementing the New Deal in order to eliminate inappropriate duties were set against a backdrop of financial constraint and a developing purchaser and provider culture. Innovative strategies to reduce hours and eliminate inappropriate duties for junior doctors were devolved to local task groups in hospital trusts. These groups were charged with effecting new ways of working and encouraging others to take on new responsibilities. Power factors came into play within the negotiations, with the task groups led by medical staff in the main, supported by chief executives and human resource staff. Nurses, who were expected to take on many of the inappropriate duties, were often not included in the negotiations or were consulted at a very late stage in the deliberations. Although nurse practitioners and clinical nurse specialists were to be involved in the implementation of the new ways of working (developing phlebotomy services, setting up new admission units), they had limited or no influence in the negotiation process.

Discussion

The changes that resulted were brought in under the guise of expanding responsibilities or extending roles, with nurse leaders often marginalised in any negotiations that took place (Palmer & Wilson 1997). As a result of this non-negotiation and imbalance of power at a critical stage of the NHS changes, the duties deemed inappropriate for junior doctors were passed on as appropriate for nursing staff beginning to be affected by recruitment and retention problems. The changes were imposed on an increasingly beleaguered workforce, without effective discussion and in many instances no increase in remuneration. If such a situation is to be prevented in the future it is important that nurse managers and leaders engage actively in the early stages of any negotiations and forcefully present their case. This is particularly important where others have a formidable power base (Traynor 1999).

Influencing and negotiating skills

THE FRAMEWORK FOR SUCCESSFUL NEGOTIATION

In identifying a framework for successful negotiation in practice it is helpful initially to consider the aspects that you need to reflect on as you seek to negotiate. The phases of preparation, orchestration and evaluation as they apply to negotiation will now be explored. A series of reflective questions are identified to allow you to relate to any previous experiences that you have had to help you think about how you will perform during negotiations to achieve your required outcomes. The first phase of the negotiation process should involve adequate preparation.

Preparation

Preparation concerns those aspects that will assist you in getting ready to make your case and commence the activities that will help you set the scene and influence the outcome of negotiations. In essence, this is about ensuring that you are prepared to enter the negotiations and that you have developed a clear strategy or plan of action. To achieve effective negotiations, it is important to appreciate and understand what Engel (1996) calls the process of negotiation which involves recognising the many factors that influence each negotiation. Such factors may be varied but often concern the nature of the relationship of the negotiating parties, the financial situation, any previous negotiations and who has the power and authority to enter into the negotiations. Engel (1996) also recommends that in attempting any negotiation you should identify and appreciate the history between the negotiating individuals or parties, the context for the negotiation, the expectations that surround the negotiations and any other external factors that may be brought to bear on the negotiating process. This is turn will assist you in becoming aware of the culture or climate in which the negotiations are to occur.

As a nurse manager, you may be negotiating individually with someone from your own profession or with another member of a different profession or occupational group. You may also be negotiating on behalf of others or within a team, in discussion with another team. In determining the context of the negotiations you should consider what you want to achieve and you need to ask yourself the following.

- What is the reason for the negotiation?
- What or who is driving the negotiations?

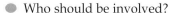

- Who should be involved?
- How am I intending to influence others?
- What new relationships do I need to develop?
- What resources can I draw on?

In answering these questions you will get a clear focus of the starting point for your negotiations and why you are engaging in the process. They also fit well with Weightman's (1996) view in determining a set of questions that will illuminate your intentions and those of others engaged in the process. She suggests that you consider:

- What do I want from the negotiations?
- What do I imagine the other individual/side wants?

These two questions are asking you to consider what your aim, goal or objectives are for the negotiation being contemplated.

The result of these reflections will become important as you engage in the initial discussions to set the scene and work towards influencing the views of others and gaining consensus. Weightman (1996) and others recommend that having a clear aim or intention will allow you to focus on the issues and is a common factor in determining success (Hiltrop & Udall 1995). Asking these sorts of reflective questions and examining your responses helps in clarifying your intentions for the process and better prepares you for any eventualities that may arise during negotiations. The responses you give will put you in a good position to set a realistic offer and avoid giving away concessions or weakening your case.

Negotiation history

Case study 3.3   The impact of a previous history

Consider Carol, a new nurse manager in a busy surgical unit comprising four wards. She is keen to use her developing management skills to do a good job in her first senior post in a new hospital. Following a recent review and an activity analysis which has demonstrated the need to change working practices, she has decided to set up a working party to help her negotiate the necessary changes. This working party involves two of the ward managers, a clinical nurse specialist and two other committed staff members. After 3 months Carol is both surprised and disappointed to realise that her working party is not working, nothing is being achieved and she is experiencing a hard time. More worryingly, as she confides to a senior colleague, her plans are being unravelled and ward staff are becoming increasingly confrontational.

Case study 3.3 (*Cont.*)

In discussing Carol's arrangements her colleague identifies, without being told, the particular member of the working party who is being disruptive and who appears to be at the centre of the unravelling of ideas and activities. Carol is very surprised to learn that the difficult group member twice applied for the post that Carol now has and was turned down each time. This person wanted to leave following the second interview but she was persuaded to stay on because the Director of Nursing Services suggested she could act up and provide stability until the new manager arrived. Carol was suddenly acutely aware of where her main difficulties lay and quickly set about building relationships and reorganising her working party.

The history between negotiating individuals and parties is important because it can impact positively or negatively on events and appreciating historical influences allows you to manage events (the orchestrating aspect of the negotiations) more meaningfully. These relationships and the issues that emerge need also to be considered within this preparatory phase. You should ask yourself the following questions.

● What do I know about who I am negotiating with?
● What is the history between us?
● If there is no previous history then ask yourself the question – what can I discover about the other party?
● If there is a history of negotiation and previous exchanges have occurred then you should ask – what was our involvement or the outcome?

When considering who you are negotiating with it is important that you uncover any history concerning those involved and explore the nature of any relationships that exist. In considering Case studies 3.1 and 3.3, it becomes apparent that there is a history to the current complex negotiations. In Case study 3.1, discussions in the past have not always gone smoothly, resulting in strikes by the workers and hard-hitting press releases by the management. Each side, both management and unions, is influenced by their own perspectives on how to handle the current situation and by the history that exists between them. This is evidenced by the communications in the media with management stressing the need for increased productivity, value for money and a drive for efficiency. The unions are keen to communicate to the commuting public that this effectively means redundancies and job losses. The unions are also stressing the case for passenger safety and the need for more guards on trains. Both sides are committed to achieving a better

Personal communication

service for passengers but a history of tension, one-day strikes and downsizing operations gives rise to the perception, on both sides, of broken promises, producing factors that will affect the current negotiations. In Case study 3.3 the disabling working party member appears to be carrying a grudge and needs help to work through the previous history to allow her to make a more enabling contribution to the management of the changes.

Determining the previous history and the factors that will impinge on the negotiations, along with a consideration of who you are negotiating with, will help you to determine the context for the negotiation.

The context of negotiations

The context of the negotiations concerns the characters and personalities involved, time pressures and the activities of others not directly involved in the negotiations. The type of culture that exists within the organisation also affects the context of the negotiations. It is evident that a culture that promotes individual respect, open dialogue and transparency in systems and procedures will encourage a similar environment for the negotiations.

Consider the company 3M, where the culture is one of creativity and healthy competition and the organisation is one where employees are valued and rewarded. 3M actively involves its staff in all stages of the design process (Mitchell 1991). The staff are seen as valuable members of the organisation who are encouraged to share their ideas and in return are rewarded for their endeavours. The organisational culture encourages problem solving and creative thinking which in turn motivates staff. Imagine the type of negotiating process that would take place in such an organisation and contrast this with your own situation, by reflecting on the following.

- What is the culture of my organisation?
- What external factors would impede any negotiations I undertake?
- What external factors would ensure successful negotiations?

The culture of an organisation will impact on the nature of any negotiations and it is evident that if we are to encourage a culture of open dialogue and mutual respect in the NHS, we need to stimulate healthy negotiations and general debate (Palmer 2001). As others have identified, negotiations do not happen in a vacuum (Engel 1996) and creating an atmosphere of collaboration and co-operation that allows individuals to thrash out the salient issues

Influencing and negotiating skills

and discover each other's point of view will promote a context for negotiations that is beneficial and will achieve results.

Having a clear idea of the context for the negotiations also allows you to begin to consider the second phase in the proposed negotiation framework which involves orchestration or managing the negotiation events.

Orchestration

Orchestration is where you discover your negotiating style, manage the actual events of the negotiation and apply your influencing and persuading skills effectively to obtain your goals. This phase should begin with a careful consideration of each individual's or each side's expectations. In illuminating the expectations that may impact on the negotiating process, it is important to think about the following points.

- What expectations do I have about the negotiations?
- What are my perceptions based on (real or perceived, factual or intuitive)?
- What could the other side's expectations be?
- What is my expectation of the negotiating environment?

Exploring your and others' expectations in this way will give you some idea of the position of each party and whether the environment will be honest, hostile, manipulative or facilitative. This orchestration stage will also be affected by the context in which the negotiations are set. This includes your previous experience as well as your communicative capabilities (Fig. 3.2). Considering the communicative skills you possess also allows you to identify and work on your particular presentation style that you will then maintain during the negotiations. A style or negotiation approach is a convenient way of presenting a collection of behaviours under one overall heading. It is, as Honey (1988) suggests, a useful shorthand for various bits and pieces of behaviour that, taken together, give a demonstrable pattern. A key facet of effective negotiation is that you feel comfortable with your style.

Identifying your style

It is important to consider what style you have developed or intend developing during the negotiations because you should feel comfortable with your approach. This will give you confidence which will be conveyed to those you are negotiating with. It is important to note that if you are not sure of your style or feel uncomfortable

Personal communication

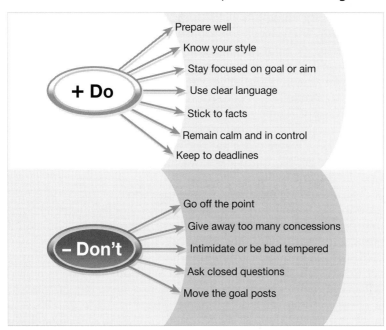

Figure 3.2 Factors to consider in presenting your case.

with it, this may be misinterpreted during negotiations. This is also true if you try to adopt a style that does not fit with your general personality as this will make you feel ill at ease which would be counter-productive as you make your case.

A useful principle is to develop a style that you feel happy with and one that can be sustained during the period of the negotiations. Inconsistencies in style or approach will confuse those you are negotiating with and may lead to mixed messages as you communicate. It will certainly affect the atmosphere of the discussions and may not encourage openness and honesty, where trust and respect can be built between the negotiating partners.

In identifying your personal negotiating style you need to consider how best to make your case clearly and effectively in a manner that allows you to marshall your thoughts, think creatively and respond to rigorous argument. In order to determine your preferred style you should consider questions such as the following.

- How do I want to come across?
- How will I maintain the focus for the discussions?
- How will I get my main points across?
- How can I be clear in what I want to say?
- How can I push for what I believe in?

Questions like these will help you to explore your personal style which may have developed from your engagement in previous negotiations or from observing the interactions of others during negotiations. If you are negotiating formally for the first time at work, you should draw on your experiences in chairing meetings, discussing issues with colleagues or taking part in clinical supervision sessions. These are effective situations where relevant communication skills are utilised regularly. You may have been fortunate to have had a mentor who has encouraged you to develop a questioning and critical approach to how you operate at work (Morton-Cooper & Palmer 2000).

You should also draw on your experiences of any formal programmes of learning or staff development that may have covered interpersonal or presentation skills. Less formally, you could check out with colleagues and seek feedback about how you come across. Remember, the important aspect here is to discover your own style and to feel safe with it to ensure that you maintain your confidence during the negotiations. As stated previously, adopting a style that does not fit your character never really works and will certainly impede the negotiation process at some point.

The various styles that work well during negotiations are those that are:

- persuasive
- analytical
- assertive
- idealistic

or a mixture of all of these.

These styles, as well as matching your personality, should also fit with the context and climate of the negotiations. In the corporate world, it is likely that 'aggressive' would be added to the list (Engel 1996) but you need to think about whether such a style would suit your needs and would work in your organisation. In business, an aggressive style may be welcomed and be viewed as a strong, forceful stance in making a case. However, in other more vocationally orientated environments, this style may be perceived as defensive and destructive. This does not mean that you should never use aggression during negotiations but it should be used sparingly, considering how it will impact on the negotiating parties and the final outcome.

Once you have identified your style you will be attempting to get your message across or make your case to get the agreement required.

Personal communication

Making your case

Here you are presenting your view and it is important to remain focused and be clear about what your intentions are. In addition, it is essential to make sure that the other side clearly hears your view. In the preparation phase you will have identified your goals or aims but you also need to have identified what is negotiable and what is not. Just as importantly, you need to have considered what to give up and when you should do this. During the exchanges you need to listen actively by paying close attention to what is going on. When asking key questions you need to maintain a calm tone and be persistent, always coming back to your main focus to reinforce your argument.

These pointers will help you communicate clearly about what you want and what you are offering in return. In this type of exchange it is helpful to have prepared yourself fully and to have attempted to visualise the exchanges (Fowler 1996). During these exchanges you also need to be aware of your body language and non-verbal communication, as discussed elsewhere in this book. To make your case clearly you should:

- remain focused on your goals and aims
- strengthen your position by focusing on facts
- attack the issue, not the person
- use clear straightforward language, avoiding exaggeration or ambiguity
- avoid going off the point
- disagree constructively
- allow the other person or side to be heard
- keep any deadlines
- know when to quit.

Other considerations concern how you present the facts and ensure that everyone involved gets the same message (Hattersley & McJannet 1997). You will probably be making a verbal presentation and should make relevant notes to help you keep on track. Increasingly information technology is being used by those engaged in the negotiation process. Computer packages such as PowerPoint make it easier for the novice presenter to get their message across in a professional manner. Once again, the important factor here is to use a medium that you feel comfortable with and can control with confidence.

Overhead transparencies and well-constructed handouts are helpful in making a point or offering clarity in getting your message across. Here, a useful way to build self-confidence is to

Influencing and negotiating skills

63

rehearse your argument with others to obtain constructive feedback. This will help to modify your deliberations. Being clear about what you want and how best to present this will be beneficial and will help to prevent mistakes being made during your negotiations. What you do not want is for the negotiations to fail.

Why negotiations fail

In considering why negotiations fail, Hiltrop & Udall (1995) build on the work of Illich (1992) to offer a comprehensive list of the mistakes that managers make during negotiations. Common errors include:

- entering negotiations with your mind made up
- not knowing who has the final negotiating authority
- failing to produce substantial arguments
- giving up too early when negotiations are blocked
- losing control over non-essential factors
- not knowing when to close the bargain.

Kennedy et al (1987) identify a series of common avoidable mistakes and in the preparation phase, these involve having unspecified aims, a weak strategy or a badly defined fall-back position. The mistakes made during the orchestration phase are varied and some overlap with what Illich (1992) identified. Avoidable mistakes include:

- opening with an unrealistic offer
- failing to state your conditions
- giving away concessions and weakening your position
- complaining, not proposing
- using weak language such as 'I'd like', 'we wish', etc.
- behaving inconsistently/moving the goal posts
- asking closed questions
- not actively listening
- arguing for the sake of it and scoring unnecessary points
- the inability to stop bargaining.

Having managed the negotiations successfully and avoided the common errors, you can begin to contemplate the third and final phase of the negotiation framework. This is where you evaluate the negotiation process and it is the stage where you are expected to record and critically reflect on what has occurred.

Evaluation

This is a key aspect of any negotiation because an effective evaluation will assist you in making preparations for your next negotiation. Any evaluation should ensure that you review and reflect on what went on, what was achieved and what determined the successful outcome or not, as the case may be. In this stage of the process you need to engage in what Thomson (1996) defines as critical reasoning. This is where you are required to think clearly, gather appropriate evidence and critically analyse and evaluate your own and others' abilities.

In the evaluation phase it is important to make notes of the meetings, summarise the main points and identify clearly the issues that emerged. It is important to keep accurate notes and add to them regularly during the process as this will give you more to work with when the negotiations are complete. Being thorough at this stage will assist with future negotiations and aid your learning. The evaluative questions are as follows.

- What went well?
- What did not go well?
- What would I do differently next time?
- What did I learn?
- How will this learning impact on any future negotiation?

Practice checklist

- Always remember that negotiation involves at least two individuals working together to reach an agreement to change something or make progress.
- Persuasion is an integral element of effective negotiation.
- It is only possible to achieve everything you want in an ideal world and, in reality, negotiation will involve some compromise.
- Negotiation can be broken down into four components:
  - concilliation
  - concession
  - compromise and
  - consensus.
- Before engaging in negotiation it is important to prepare thoroughly. Aim to be informed and understand the history and context of the situation within which you are negotiating and be aware of any fall-back positions you may wish to adopt.

Influencing and negotiating skills

Practice checklist (*Cont.*)

● Aim to identify your own style of negotiation and become comfortable and familiar with it to maximise your effectiveness when involved in a situation where negotiation is necessary.
● Try to develop an appreciation of why some negotiations fail and use what you learn from this to improve your own practice.

Discussion questions

● Try to recall from your own experience situations where negotiations you have experienced have failed or succeeded. What do you think influenced the outcome of these negotiations?
● Within your area of work or responsibility, try to list issues on which you would wish to negotiate. Which of these would be a priority? Can you predict areas of success and failure?
● Using examples from your own clinical experience or from a service environment around you, can you identify aspects of culture and the service content which would militate against successful negotiation or influence the possibility of a successful outcome?

CONCLUSION

Making sure that you are well prepared, adept at making your case and engaging in a thorough evaluation should help you become a successful negotiator and one who looks forward to future negotiations with confidence. I end with the words of a president who negotiated his country from the brink of a potential world war following the Cuban missile crisis in the early 1960s.

> Let us never negotiate out of fear. But never let us fear to negotiate.
> (JF Kennedy 1961)

References

Barr H 1996 Ends and means in interprofessional education. Education for Health 9(3): 341–352

Barr H 2001 Working effectively together. Overcoming the barriers. MAPE Conference, Oulu, Finland. 10 May 2001

Carpenter J 1995 Doctors and nurses: stereotypes and stereotype change in interprofessional education. Journal of Interprofessional Care 9(2): 151–161

Clampitt PG 1991 Communicating for managerial effectiveness. Sage Publications, California

Cleeton D, Sharman D 2000 Influencing skills. Fenman, London

Davies C 1995 Gender and the professional predicament in nursing. Open University Press, Buckingham

Department of Health 1991 New deal on junior doctors' hours. HMSO, London

Department of Health 2000 A health service of all the talents: developing the NHS workforce. DoH, London

Engel PH 1996 Negotiating. McGraw-Hill, New York

Fowler A 1996 Negotiation skills and strategies, 2nd edn. Institute of Personnel Development, London

Hattersley ME, McJannet LM 1997 Management communication. Principles and practice. McGraw-Hill, Columbus, Ohio

Hiltrop JM, Udall S 1995 The essence of negotiation. Prentice-Hall, London

Honey P 1988 Improve your people skills. Institute of Personnel Management, London

Illich J 1992 Deal-breakers and breakthroughs. Wiley, New York

Kennedy G, Benson J, McMillan J 1987 Managing negotiations. How to get a better deal, 3rd edn. Hutchinson Business, London

Klein R 1989 The politics of the NHS, 2nd edn. Longman, London

Meads G, Ashcroft J 2000 Relationships in the NHS. Bridging the gap. Royal Society of Medicine Press, London

Metropolitan Police Service 2000 Policing London: the MPS Report and Plans 2000. MPS, London

Mitchell R 1991 Masters of innovation: how 3M keeps its new products coming. In: Henry J, Walker D (eds) Managing innovation. Sage Publications, London

Morton-Cooper A, Palmer A 2000 Mentoring, preceptorship and clinical supervision. A guide to professional support roles in practice. Blackwell Science, Oxford

Obholzer A, Roberts VZ (eds) 1994 The unconscious at work. Individual and organisational stress in the human services. Routledge, London

Palmer A 2001 Freedom to learn, freedom to be: learning: reflecting and supporting in practice. In: Humphris D, Masterson A (eds) Developing new clinical roles. A guide for health professionals. Churchill Livingstone, London

Palmer A, Wilson A 1997 New deal: new directions – the evaluation of 'innovations in practice projects'. South Thames NHS Executive, London

Pennington DC 2001 The social psychology of small groups. Taylor and Francis, London

Peplau HE 1952 Interprofessional relations in nursing. Palgrave, London

Thomson A 1996 Critical reasoning. A practical introduction. Routledge, London

Influencing and negotiating skills

Tovey P (ed) 2000 Contemporary primary care. The challenges of change. Open University Press, Buckingham

Traynor M 1999 Managerialism and nursing. Beyond oppression and profession. Routledge, London

Weightman J 1996 Managing people in the health service. Institute of Personnel Development, London

Wicks D 1998 Nurses and doctors at work: rethinking professional boundaries. Open University Press, Buckingham

Wolfe B 1990 Friendly persuasion: how to negotiate and win. Berkley Books, New York

Further reading

Back K, Back K 1999 Assertiveness at work: a practical guide to handling awkward situations. McGraw-Hill, London

Emap Healthcare 2000 NT open learning: the complexity of human interaction. Nursing Times 97(13): 45–48

Johnson S 1998 Who moved my cheese? An amazing way to deal with change in your work and in your life. Vermilion, London

McCormack MH 1995 On negotiating. Dane Books, Beverly Hills, California

Personal communication

Application 3:1

Mark Darley

Negotiation: advice and support from a health trade union

The health union Unison has a comprehensive website (www.unison.org.uk) providing a range of news, information and advice for members and anyone accessing the site, aimed at nurses and other health care workers in need of advice and support faced with situations in which they may need to negotiate. This could be for clinically based staff or those with increasing managerial responsibilities.

The area on the site that deals with 'bargaining' is relevant to the subject matter dealt with in Chapter Three. The range of fact sheets that can be displayed and printed for the August 2001 update include such diverse issues as:

- current UNISON pay settlements
- parental leave and time off
- performance-related pay
- teachers, police and civil service
- working time – hours and holidays
- management consultants
- private contractors – second report
- provision of education services by the private sector
- annual leave
- bargaining with company accounts.

In addition to newsletters packed with information on health-related matters, these provide the type of information that many health care professionals require to negotiate their position or act with better understanding of issues affecting them, their colleagues and patient welfare. One aspect of the use of modern technology to support health professionals is the inclusion of an email address for the Bargaining Support Group.

It is also interesting to note that the website provides the latest information on European legislation and its impact on the work of the NHS. When the usual confusion that surrounds such legislation is taken into account it is easy to see how this type of information and support can be invaluable to a clinical professional engaged in negotiation to influence conditions in the clinical area. The key point here is that negotiation and bargaining, as a trade union might refer to it, is heavily dependent on accurate and up-to-date information. Use of the ever-increasing amount of information on the World Wide Web suggests that clinical professionals engaged in negotiation can no longer feel uninformed on the vital issues of the day and how they impact on their everyday work and the way they care for patients.

Other professional bodies such as the RCN, UKCC (Nursing and Midwifery Council from April 2002), the four National Boards for Nursing, Midwifery and Health Visiting and the Department of Health, as well as trade unions representing other clinical groups, provide similar websites and information services. While the skills required to negotiate and influence people and situations need to be developed at a personal level, access to information to support these skills has never been more readily available.

Chapter **Four**

Marketing yourself, the profession and the organisation

Yvonne Hill, Helen Brett

- Historical influences perpetuating stereotypes
- Gender
- Professionalism redefined
- Marketing yourself
- Understanding the meaning of self

- Developing your sense of self
- Organisations
- Organisational culture
- Suggested ways for becoming a more effective leader

O V E R V I E W

Communication is the most important and arguably the most critical skill in management and leadership as everything that a manager does in some way influences the actions of others. It follows therefore that the impact of any manager's communication has far-reaching consequences beyond their immediate audience as judgements may not only be made of them as individuals but also about both the profession to which they belong and the organisation they serve. It is therefore evident that to be effective in this role, managers need to use strategies that will help them to accomplish not only the goals and objectives of their organisation but also to motivate their staff to join them in this endeavour. Just as governments may be judged by the performance of one or two of their members so too will the public's perception of an organisation be influenced by the behaviour of individuals working within it. Think how often you have judged an organisation just by the actions of one employee talking to you on the telephone!

Personal communication

INTRODUCTION

This chapter discusses the historical influences which have affected the way in which effective communication in nursing in particular has been impeded. It goes on to identify ways in which health care professionals can overcome these influences to develop and utilise appropriate 'marketing' strategies within their organisations. This will necessitate an appraisal of self and the ability to inspire, support and empower others. Nursing provides an excellent example of how a profession, in spite of its numerical strength, has often failed to communicate within the health care system, leading to disempowerment of its members in the eyes of many.

Finally, use of the term 'marketing' might seem strange and out of place to some readers but the term in its descriptive sense is helpful in stating what health care professionals need to do to get their point across. Outside professional groups, a well-understood or accepted issue may not receive a similarly positive response in other arenas. In the broader sense, we are always engaged in some form of marketing when speaking or working outside our professional groups. What is said and how a person comes across reinforce either positive or negative views of the individual and often the profession they are in.

HISTORICAL INFLUENCES PERPETUATING STEREOTYPES

Many health care professions outside medicine can argue that stereotypes often define their approach to clinical work, especially teamwork. This is particularly so for the numerically dominant nursing profession. Barker et al (1995) claimed that nursing was 'socially constructed' not only by its history but also its subsequent inability to control its own destiny. Ideas such as passivity, obedience and subservience have long been associated with the socialisation of nurses and unfortunately, are still current today. But these are directly opposed to the notions of autonomy, self-control and self-regulation which are deemed to be the fundamental requirements of an emerging profession, striving for recognition. Equally they may also stifle creative decision making and problem solving and thus are likely, in turn, to affect the real and perceived status of the nurse.

Davies (1996) felt that it is precisely because the profession has clung to the revered traditions and rituals of nursing that its development has been hampered. Because of this, she felt that the doctor has come to be regarded as the 'natural' and senior decision maker in all aspects of health care, mostly at nurses' expense. Many in other health care professions could argue a similar point, though with differing perceptions of the impact on their professional development This then verifies to public onlookers that nothing has changed and even though individual, innovative nurses may be struggling to raise the image of the profession through such activities as research, participation in policy making at local and national level and continual updating, according to Cavanagh (1991) most nurses are still failing to deal constructively or resolutely with these overarching issues.

GENDER

Gender issues have, seemingly, also played a part in holding back nurses, and in particular managers, from developing their full potential. Even now nursing is predominantly a female profession. The 'good' nurse was mostly portrayed as gentle, patient, kind and devoted (Savage 1985) and as women's work has tended to be undervalued by society, so has the status and image of nursing. With approximately 95% of the nursing workforce still female, Davies (1995) argued that because women have been regarded as weak, irrational, emotional and passive as opposed to men being seen as strong, rational and active, this has hindered them from occupying the higher paid positions that males currently enjoy. It would seem, therefore, that female managers still have additional hurdles to overcome before they are accepted as equals within an organisation.

Patriarchal practices (Hartmann 1976) which attempt to explain the power base of men and women and the consequent male-dominated control have tended to leave women in relatively powerless positions and their resistance has been disorganised and ineffective. Fitzgerald (1990) also believed that female nurses have taken a subservient role within the health care system for too long and if they continue to believe that this is the proper order then very little will change. Irigararay (1993) argued that ignoring these differences did little to empower women and actually perpetuated the male-dominated world. But equally, women have hindered their own development by assuming that the male model was the only successful one.

Marketing Yourself, the profession and the organisation

With these existing stereotypes, nurses, and in particular managers, need to consider the most effective way to move forward. Whilst Witz (1992) acknowledged that nurses could exert more influence on others if they all bargained with one voice and demanded a greater say in how they were employed, Rushing (1993) stated that before this could be achieved, they would have to clarify their own ideology and persuade society of nursing's unique contribution.

PROFESSIONALISM REDEFINED

Perhaps we will need to adopt the new model of professionalism, proposed by Davies (1995), which advocates replacing the outmoded, restrictive, arrogant and inward-looking concept of profession with a power-sharing model, emphasising engagement, the use of self in interactions and interpersonal expertise. Professionalism, as she terms it, appears to be an amalgam of both the objective and subjective or technical and interpersonal expertise which is needed to inform contemporary practice. Gavin (1997) argued that the essence of professionalism is expertise and how this is operationalised yet the degree to which nursing is recognised as a profession has been debated both inside and outside nursing. The relocation of nursing education into the higher education sector and the development of a body of nursing knowledge through research have gone some way to improving the image and status of the profession. Castledine (1998) argued that nurses must be orientated to the beliefs, values and attitudes expected of members of a profession before they could either adopt ideals or move on.

As early as 1981, Cohen identified that the nursing culture itself was an impediment to adopting a professional stance. She argued that even during their education, students received contradictory messages about how they should behave. For example, on the one hand they were encouraged to be questioning, challenging of other professionals and fully accountable for their actions while on the other, were required to be obedient and adopt near-perfect, stereotypical images from the past. Perhaps the 'ghost of the Crimea' still influences us! Even today, nurses who adopt entrepreneurial and innovative approaches to client care can meet with strong opposition. For example, Baraniak (Dinsdale 1998) found that during the initial stages of setting up a nurse-led clinic within a general practice setting, some of the local GPs did not consider it to be a serious endeavour and 'laughed in her face'. But she persisted as she had

Personal communication

sufficient courage, energy and self-belief to overcome some of their rigidly held views. Huber (1996) suggested that it is how nurses value themselves that ultimately affects the way others perceive them. So, if we do not value our profession then it is unlikely that others will. Goward (1992) reminds us that we should not discard all our historical images as society still values us as we are, even though the professional status of others appears to have diminished our own (Aber & Hawkins 1992).

The image that managers need to project is therefore one of competence, authority, professionalism, confidence and wisdom. Porter (1992) found that an individual's positive self-perception and effectiveness increased with knowledge. Even though physicians still have power advantages, senior nurses are able to contribute to professional decision making in increasingly effective ways. It follows, then, that marketing the profession of nursing will be easier if we possess a strong knowledge and power base and a positive self-image and temper this with respect for others. The values and beliefs of nursing need to be communicated to others in a purposeful and enthusiastic way.

MARKETING YOURSELF

As understanding ourselves is very complex and there are parts of us which we are reluctant to share with others, it would be helpful if the reader could identify the following in both an honest and constructive way.

- How satisfied are you with yourself?
- How much of your real self do you show to other people?
- How do others view you?

Of course, we can never be quite sure how others view us but usually there are indications which may give us some insight into our own performance.

UNDERSTANDING THE MEANING OF SELF

It is also useful to remember that there are three aspects of self.

- *Our perceived self* – this covers not only what we are but also our social status such as job and salary and religion and/or ethnic group.
- *Our desired self* – this is the one which we try to attain and might concern our job, qualification or even partner.

75

● *Our third self* – this is the one which we want to project to the outside world. Whilst this could be the same as the perceived self, they can sometimes be at odds with each other and thus cause us to send out conflicting messages to others.

Adler (1994) suggests that there is a strong link between self, behaviour and communication. For example, if you are nervous when dealing with those in authority you may be more likely to adopt diffident behaviour. People often blush or stumble over their words when they are ill at ease. This in turn may encourage a negative response from others and could result in the person feeling more vulnerable and insecure. However, if you adopt a more assertive approach, you are more likely to gain a positive response which in turn is likely to affect the way others view you but, perhaps more importantly, ultimately how you view yourself. It is logical to suppose that a confident, self-assured person will gain the trust and support of others more easily than an ill-at-ease and nervy person.

Henry Ford's saying is therefore very apt:

If you think you can or can't, you are right.

DEVELOPING YOUR SENSE OF SELF

Having examined the notion of self-concept and its effect on behaviour and communication, the next section is intended to help you improve your self-image by thinking about the following.

Don't be too hard on yourself – be realistic

You may have set your goals too high and find that they are impossible to reach. Try to have realistic expectations of your own performance and focus on the things which you do well. Seek out people who will value your contribution, not in an uncritical way but who view you positively.

Be ready and willing to change

This will require flexibility, effort and being open to criticism without becoming defensive. Really believe that you can change.

Develop skills to present a good image

You might start by seeking advice from friends, colleagues or a mentor but a word of caution here; the advice you receive may not be what you want to hear or be very helpful. Secondly, whilst seeking advice from books can be worthwhile and give you some practical examples to follow, they will not be able to provide feedback. The important thing is that you experience different techniques and see how they work for you.

Your image may be enhanced by these simple, yet effective actions which you could try.

- Wear a jacket, especially when you want to make an impact.
- Hold your head up.
- Prepare well before and speak confidently at a meeting; this is essential if you are to have a positive effect on both yourself and your audience.
- Write what you want to say on a card before a meeting/interview if you have difficulty in identifying what you need to say and also if you are unable to express yourself clearly.
- Learn from positive role models – watch how they act and behave. This may also demystify the process for you and enable you to realise that you can also act in this way!

Finally you need to appreciate that your self-concept has an enormous effect on the way you communicate and how others judge you. But even though you can recognise this, it may still be difficult to change as many of our attitudes and behaviours were shaped in early childhood.

These self-development issues are developed further in Chapters Two and Six.

But it can be done?

It is now necessary to look at how you can further develop yourself. This will enable you to develop a professional and empowering managerial stance within your organisation. The relevant literature is far from clear on whether managers need to be leaders. There seems to be some consensus (Alimo-Metcalfe 1996, Antrobus 1998, Marquis & Huston 1996) that managers with limited leadership abilities tend to focus on controlling tasks whereas those who have developed enhanced skills do empower others much more effectively. As empowerment of others is seen to be crucial in the context of promoting the organisation and the profession of nursing, it would seem that managers do require these special skills.

Whilst Antrobus (1998) defined a leader as someone with a sense of purpose and integrity, ability to motivate, inspire and also facilitate change in others, Fiedler & Garcia (1987) stressed that,

Marketing Yourself, the profession and the organisation

more importantly, it was these characteristics that determined not only the success of but the very survival of the organisation.

Within the many definitions of leadership two major themes have emerged. They are concerned with the ability to interact with and at the same time influence others. Huber (1996, p.51) defined leadership as 'the process of influencing people to accomplish goals' which considerably moves on from Bennis' (1994) definition which only advocates that a manager is 'a person who focuses more on systems and administration rather than on innovation within the workplace'.

In reality both roles often overlap yet it would be unwise to assume that managers necessarily make good leaders. Leadership abilities, used wisely, can confer empowerment which enables others to use their own innate or learned skills authoritatively, which in turn increases their responsibility and belief in their own powers. Leaders, however, cannot do this alone as they require their followers to share the same vision before they can combine their talents and promote their organisation and profession. Empowering others, therefore, is seen as a critical feature of shared governance. This, according to Porter-O'Grady (1989), shares power, control and autonomy which ultimately should result in everyone adopting appropriate professional behaviour.

Empowering others requires managers/leaders to be effective communicators. Managers need to develop or possess the ability to be self-aware and cognisant of both their strengths and weaknesses. Wright (1995) believes that leaders should be assertive without being aggressive. They need to use their hearts as well as their heads and combine both masculine traits, such as power, with the female, sensitive ones. He lists a number of desirable attributes for a leader:

- consistency
- sense of humour
- strong sense of justice
- clarity of thought
- inspirational and energising abilities
- unafraid to display compassion and caring.

Leadership styles

Markham (1996) maintained that there has been a fundamental shift away from traditional models of management based on hierarchical approaches to ones which are more subtle. This involved crossing organisational boundaries and using personal influence as the main tool. She proposes that the two styles of leadership based on Rosener's (1990) work could be adopted within the workforce. These developmental models are transactional and transformational and are set out in Box 4.1.

The transformational style appears to encompass many of the qualities which nurse managers should possess so that they can promote both themselves and their organisation. It provides a broader perspective that takes into account some of the complexities of organisational culture. Burns (1978) suggests that transformational leaders engage with others in such a way that the leader's and the followers' aspirations merge. This relationship allows this by raising the 'level of human conduct and ethical aspiration of both leader and led' (Burns 1978, p.20).

Transforming leadership thus shapes and alters the goals in order to achieve a common purpose and through this style managers are not only committed to their own promotion of the organisation but facilitate others to do the same.

We have identified the need for nurse managers to be good leaders in order to market themselves and the organisation and we suggest that a transformational style is the most effective. Encompassed within the model are visibility, flexibility, authority, assistance and giving constructive feedback. We could add further qualities of risk taking, courage and the ability to work efficiently and effectively. Positive leadership can make an enormous difference to the working climate and to everyone who works in it. In an increasingly changing environment, nurses are likely to function better if they have a leader who has clear goals which all staff are familiar with and committed to and especially that their efforts are recognised and acknowledged when they

---

Box 4.1   Leadership styles

Transactional leadership style Dunham & Klafehn (1990)	*Transformational leadership style* Klakovich (1994) Marriner-Tomey (1993)
Rewards and punishment for performance Uses power that comes from organisational position and formal authority	Collaboration Ascribing power to interpersonal skills and personal contact Consensus seeking Consultative Strong personal ethic Empowering Hardiness

Marketing Yourself, the profession and the organisation

achieve them. Well-motivated staff are likely to promote their organisation and profession more positively than staff who are discontented!

ORGANISATIONS

Organisations are about structure, purpose and people (Fig. 4.1). How these interact with each other will determine an organisation's character and nature. Organisational values have changed over the past few years and many are now different from the ones that managers and others were taught when they first entered their career pathways. It seems that whilst the hierarchy has established and embraced different values these may not have filtered down to the 'shop floor.' Or as Sams (1998) dares to suggest, these nurses may not have been motivated enough to find out or just felt too intimidated by senior managers to ask. The introduction of the 'more academic' nurse through the Project 2000 initiative, the demise of the traditional 'hands-on carer' and the introduction of short-term contracts may have also made staff reluctant to see the whole organisational picture (Gutteridge 1996), as it may feed their own feelings of inadequacy.

As the working environment changes for nurses it is often less stressful to focus on the narrow perspective of one's own job. However, Huber (1996) argues that nurses will become more effective if they become more familiar with the organisation's philosophy, style and vision. It is only then that they can begin to share in the organisation's values and beliefs and communicate these effectively to others.

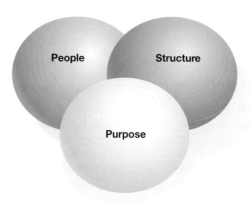

Figure 4.1   Components of an organisation.

Personal communication

ORGANISATIONAL CULTURE

Organisational culture is enormously important and serves to give its members a sense of identity. It promotes a sense of commitment and also enhances stability. The organisation's culture will be evident in the mission statement and the identified formal structure. Del Bueno & Freund (1986) identify some key elements which might tell you something about the culture of the organisation.

1. *Image* – what kind of image does the organisation portray? This might be seen in the public relations activities, its logo and other symbols and relationships with the local public and media. It is important that managers are aware of the image that the organisation is trying to convey to the outside world.
2. *Image of the employees* – how do people dress and interact with each other? What are the codes of conduct? Managers should act and dress in a way which supports this image so that there is a clear identification with the organisation and they can act as role models.
3. *Environment and ambience* – how attractive and comfortable is the environment? Has thought been given to colour schemes, space, furniture, music and fitness for purpose? These features need to be considered for both staff and the visiting public. Much attention has been paid to outpatients departments in many hospitals with a change in seating arrangements, the introduction of screens and plants and music or video recordings. An attempt has been made to reduce the strange and often austere atmosphere of hospitals. In a way the organisation is saying 'we value you as our customer and are trying to make your stay with us as comfortable as possible'. Jennings (1997) considers that nurses need to be involved in policy making as the patient or service user is now our customer. Poor publicity could result in dissatisfaction and reduced business later. Managers can be influential in decision making by knowing the right people within the organisation and being members of committees.
4. *Communication* – what are the modes and channels of communication? How well, as a manager, do you communicate with those above and below you? Is everyone treated with courtesy and respect, regardless of their position or status? How are telephone enquiries treated? Referring back to the overview, a great deal can be learned about an organisation through one phone call. That image will stay for a long time and if it is a negative one it will be difficult to change. Situations where there has been

81

perceived neglect or malpractice need to be handled very carefully as a wrong word may cause even more damage. Often, public relations consultants are employed to help organisations in these situations and those employees who have the 'right' image are selected to speak. An open, honest approach is often received most favourably.

What the leader/manager stands for and communicates to others will determine how they behave and communicate about the organisation. Building an organisational culture is based on a framework of support. Huber (1996) suggests the following guidelines for good practice.

- Start from where your employees are in their understanding.
- Adopt an open style of communication for the promotion of discussion.
- Personal contact is important. With the advent of email and other media, this is often forgotten.
- Identify a shared vision and mission so that the group knows where it is going. The group may help to shape and develop this, so that they have some ownership of the overall organisation's mission. From there the leader can help to form strategies and actions from the shared values and beliefs. Here it is important that the manager reminds the group of the overarching philosophy and that ideas are not developed in opposition to those identified by the organisation. Trust, risk taking and positive self-esteem are vital ingredients for success.
- The need for a constant examination of the group's personal values and the 'fit' with those of the organisation. A mismatch can result in conflicting values being portrayed to its members and to the outside world.
- Empowering the group by creating a work environment that values the group's choices and facilitates their investment in the organisation. Empowerment does not mean relinquishing power but is an interactive process that develops and increases power through cooperation and working together. It involves the manager allowing others to work creatively and explore different ways of doing things for the benefit of the organisation. It also will invariably mean that sometimes things go wrong; these situations need to be handled sensitively.

Effective managers need to care for themselves, present a powerful picture to others and be prepared to work hard. Marquis & Huston (1996) argue that power and energy go hand in hand. They state that it is important to:

- be visible
- keep a sense of humour
- 'blow your own trumpet'
- be flexible
- use experts.

SUGGESTED WAYS FOR BECOMING A MORE EFFECTIVE LEADER

Because nurses may not have developed the breadth of vision to appreciate an organisation's overall corporate strategy, it is vital that nurse managers acquire this ability and communicate it effectively to outsiders as well as to their individual teams. This enables them to influence those in senior positions and maintain an image of nurses that is positive and less likely to obstruct contribution to policy and practice at all levels of the organisation. Consideration and use of the points outlined in the Practice checklist open your thinking to the wider political and professional milieu which will in time allow you to make a stronger contribution to your work environment.

CONCLUSION

This chapter has focused on ways in which nurse managers can present a more positive image of themselves, their organisation and their profession through the use of more empowering models of management and leadership and being aware of the impact their communication has on others. It has also highlighted some of the constraints which influence their effectiveness and discussed strategies to overcome them. A way forward to influencing health policies at national and local level is for nursing to break free of its traditional subservient role, clarify its own ideology and persuade society of its value (Rushing 1993). It also needs to attain power through professionalism if it wishes to compete in the battle for influence in the health care system. Porter (1992) argues that professionalism will help to overcome the restricting nature of bureaucracy and management. Nurses must all contribute to the promotion of a more dynamic and positive image, with managers playing a crucial role in facilitating this.

Marketing yourself, the profession and the organisation

Personal communication

Practice checklist

- Have a working knowledge of the different leadership styles and choose styles which you feel comfortable with. Adopt different styles to suit the situation.
- Clarify your overall goals and vision for the future. Break your goals down into achievable segments.
- Communicate this to the staff with whom you work.
- Choose a mentor who can support, advise and be critical and realistic about your performance.
- Get to know the organisation well, including its strategic plans, systems and influential people within these systems. Seek their advice and support as required.
- Be aware of what is going on around you. Try not to be taken unawares by new initiatives or changes in policy.
- Identify potential obstacles or staff who are not supportive at the outset and deal with these situations appropriately.
- Make it clear what you position is and don't sit on the fence *but be prepared to be flexible.*
- Develop a communication pathway both upwards and downwards and continually evaluate it for its effectiveness.
- Listen to and give quality feedback.
- Be visible, making frequent, casual contacts with staff, but remain the authority figure. This means making and guiding any decision making but also proffering and accepting just criticism.

Discussion questions

- Identify your managerial strengths and weaknesses and consider why some are perceived to be more effective than others.
- It has been suggested that the 'nursing culture' has impeded professional development. How could you encourage a positive professional image within your organisation, in order to overcome this?
- Innovative practice inevitably involves an element of risk taking. How will you create a safe and responsive care environment using a dynamic transformational management model?
- What strategies do you use in your everyday practice to promote an empowered workforce?

References

Aber C, Hawkins J 1992 Portrayal of nurses in advertisements in medical and nursing journals. Image 24(4): 289–293

Adler RB 1994 Understanding human communication. Harcourt Brace, Philadelphia

Alimo-Metcalfe B 1996 Leaders or managers? Nursing Management 3: 22–24

Antrobus S 1998 Thoroughly modern leaders. Nursing Times 94(18): 66–67

Barker PJ, Reynolds W, Ward T 1995 The proper focus of nursing: a critique of the 'caring' ideology. International Journal of Nursing Studies 32(4): 386–397

Bennis W 1994 On becoming a leader. Addison-Wesley, Menlo Park, California

Burns JM 1978 Leadership. Harper and Row, New York

Castledine G 1998 Nursing professionalism: is it decreasing? British Journal of Nursing 7(6): 352

Cavanagh S 1991 The conflict style of nurses and managers. Journal of Advanced Nursing 16: 1254–1260

Cohen H 1981 The nurse's quest for a professional identity. Addison-Wesley, Menlo Park, California

Davies C 1995 Gender and the professional predicament in nursing. Open University, Buckingham

Davies C 1996 A new vision of professionalism. Nursing Times 92(46): 54–56

Del Bueno D, Freund C 1986 Power and politics in nursing: a casebook. National Health Publishing, Owings Mills, Maryland

Dinsdale P 1998 Pilot pioneer. Nursing Standard 12(33): 12–13

Dunham J, Klafehn K 1990 Transformational leadership and the nurse executive. Journal of Nursing Administration 20: 28–33

Fiedler F, Garcia J 1987 New approaches to effective leadership: cognitive resources and organisational performance. John Wiley, New York

Fitzgerald M 1990 Autonomy for practising nurses. Surgical Nurse 3(6): 24–26

Gavin J 1997 Nursing ideology and the 'generic care'. Journal of Advanced Nursing 26: 692–697

Goward P 1992 The development of the nursing profession. In: Kenworthy N, Snowley G, Gilling C (eds) Common foundation studies in nursing. Churchill Livingstone, Edinburgh

Gutteridge D 1996 Not at your disposal. Health Service Journal 22 Feb: 25

Hartmann H 1976 Capitalism, patriarchy and job segregation by sex. In: Giddons A, Held D (eds) Classes, power and conflict: classical and contemporary debates. Macmillan, London

Huber D 1996 Leadership and nursing care management. WB Saunders, Philadelphia

Irigararay L 1993 Je, tu, nous toward a culture of difference. Routledge, London

Jennings C 1997 The way to take charge. Nursing Times 93(42): 36–37

Klakovich M 1994 Connective leadership for the 21st century: a historical perspective and future directions. Advanced Nursing Science 16(4): 42–54

Markham G 1996 Gender in leadership. Nursing Management 3(1): 18–19

Marketing yourself, the profession and the organisation

Marquis B, Huston C 1996 Leadership roles and management functions in nursing. Lippincott, Philadelphia

Marriner-Tomey A 1993 Transformational leadership in nursing. Mosby, St Louis

Porter S 1992 The poverty of professionalism: a critical analysis of strategies for the occupational advancement of nursing. Journal of Advanced Nursing 17: 720–726

Porter-O'Grady T 1989 Shared governance: reality or sham? American Journal of Nursing 89(3): 350–351

Rosener J 1990 Ways women lead. Harvard Business Review Nov-Dec: 119–125

Rushing B 1993 Ideology in the re-emergence of North American midwifery. Work and Occupations 20(1): 46–67

Sams D 1998 When knowledge is power. Nursing Times 94(5): 77–78

Savage J 1985 The politics of nursing. Heinemann Nursing, London

Witz A 1992 Professions and patriarchy. Routledge, London

Wright S 1995 Sales pitch for nursing's softer side. Nursing Management 2(2): 16–18

Further reading

Bass BM, Avolio BJ 1994 Shatter the glass ceiling: women may make better managers. Human Resource Management Journal 33: 546–560

Bate P 1995 Strategies for cultural change. Butterworth Heinemann, London

Burnes B 1996 Managing change. Pitman Publishing, London

Cohen S, Mason D 1996 Stages of nursing's political development: where we've been and where we ought to go. Nursing Outlook 66(6): 259

Corbett J 1994 Critical cases in organisational behaviour. Macmillan, Edinburgh

Cunningham G 1997 A journey to patient-centred leadership. Royal College of Nursing, London

Mullins L 1999 Management and organisational behaviour. Financial Times and Prentice Hall, London

Trompenaars F, Hampdon-Turner C 1998 Riding the waves of culture. Nicholas Brealey, London

Personal communication

Application **4:1**

Ann P Young

The power of metaphors

Without thinking about it, we use metaphors frequently in everyday speech, to convey emotion, to make an impact, to express approval or disapproval. How much more expressive it is to say, 'I was able to spread my wings' rather than, 'I was given more scope'. To say, 'I found myself between a rock and a hard place' conveys a seemingly unresolvable conflict situation in just a few words. Being 'stabbed in the back' not only describes a negative experience but says quite a lot about the individual's attitudes to others. Metaphors provide, therefore, a very strong and powerful shorthand.

In this application, the results of a survey of 15 professional middle managers in a NHS Trust were collated on the basis of the metaphors used to describe their organisation. They were asked two specific questions.

- If you were to liken your organisation to some creature, what would that be and why?
- What should it be and why?

All but one of the managers had no difficulty in responding to the first question. Not all followed this up with a second creature as, once launched into a discussion on what was wrong with their organisation, they became verbose on what was needed to put it right! The following results for the first question will, in the main, not be a surprise – elephants were much in evidence – but the answers to the second question showed more diversity.

Typical of these managers' perceptions was a view of the organisation as slow and cumbersome, although with the potential to go faster. 'It's like a tortoise, just so slow and plodding. At times we can lift our head up and go, but then go back into our shell.' This dichotomy between retreat and advance was described as being like an ostrich. 'Bury its head in the sand and difficulties will go away – but at other times, it's go out and get it.' Two people saw the organisation as some sleeping or hibernating creature. 'But it's probably awakening from a deep sleep . . . it's started to go forward a bit now.' Similarly for the 'sleeping bear, not really exercising all the power that it has'. However, this manager also saw progress. 'I think that's less true than it was, but I still think we are a bit sleepy, yet we are a big player, one of the biggest population centres.'

A creature that is slow and lumbering was chosen by six managers: three elephants, two oxen and a sloth. The most maligned animal was the ox. 'It's a bloody ox, stubborn at times, and trying to move it is slow progress' and 'It's an ox with a limp, a big ugly creature, not knowing where it is going, and not doing it very well. It tends to lurch from one thing to another, it doesn't know where it is going, it doesn't know what it wants to do.' Similarly, the sloth was seen as 'something that moves so slowly and responds so slowly to change – I think it should wake up'.

The elephant was seen as a much more positive metaphor of the organisation. 'An elephant is slow but once it gets going, it can move although with bits flapping about a lot. Perhaps it's good that it is slow to get going as it's not too driven by what is going on around it but responds to internal drives – the balance between experience and new ideas.' To another manager, the elephant 'is large, as a body it has a long memory of its past, for better or worse, and it's lumbering along. It could go faster if it wanted to and it has a lot of potential it doesn't know it's got. We just need a bit more action. It's got immense brain power, but doesn't always use it.'

A couple of metaphors described the size and diversity of the organisation. 'It's like Topsy – that "growed and growed" ' and 'It's an octopus with lots of dangly bits. The trust has lots of fingers in lots of pies. It's chaotic.'

The two remaining metaphors were rather different. One manager was particularly concerned for her staff. 'It's a crocodile because it snaps and bites without thinking. The trust can hurt a lot of people if it's not careful, particularly employees. I've seen it. It bites off those with a lot of experience. Lots of people were retired early plus some people were made to feel uncomfortable and left.' The final metaphor illustrated the problems of communication within the trust. 'It's a giraffe, really. Its head is quite a long way from its feet. And when you look at a giraffe, its head seems to move independently of its feet, and at some time the feet follow later. And they look ungainly when they get down to the job they're supposed to be doing. To eat and reproduce, I suppose, and both are a bit ungainly! You could say a dinosaur, but it's not that. It has lots of ideas. I think the problem is communication between what could be called the top and what could be called the sharp end.'

The trawl of metaphors for what creature should typify the organisation brought greater diversity, illustrating a lack of cohesion on the image that should be presented in the marketplace. As explained, only six managers actually responded to this second question, with two cheetahs, a panda, an eagle, a dressage horse and, rather surprisingly, another elephant.

The elephant metaphor, as enlarged on above, was not presented as a totally negative image and the person who saw this for the future emphasised the positive characteristics. To her, an elephant was 'something comfortable, something strong . . . and careful with people'. The panda also represented something that was relaxed and that people could like.

The cheetah metaphor denoted an organisation that knew what it wanted and went out and got it. It was seen as quick, although taking time to look back and change direction. This was described as being a 'responsible cheetah'!

The eagle and the horse were both about visibility and showing off, although there were some differences. The organisation as an eagle would be 'more dynamic, more soaring, more up there, saying this is what we are'. There was the belief that once you had built this image, you could maintain it by 'catching the wind currents'. However, the final metaphor of the organisation as a dressage horse seemed to capture one other very important aspect of the relationship between it and its employees and users. 'It's got to be reliable and constant, to provide security for staff and patients, but I would like to see it now and again having a little stir. And being proud of what we've achieved – a bit like a dressage horse. Just now and again, I would like to see us show off a little.' Being proud of what the individual has achieved within and for that organisation seems to be a very firm base on which to build a deserved reputation.

In conclusion, perceptions colour actions. Metaphors that are purely negative may trigger positive action but it seems more likely that images that contain positive overtones along with the negative may enhance feeling good about where you work. As the last metaphor suggested, in most organisations it is possible to find some achievements of which to be proud and to use these as a basis for presenting a more positive image to those both inside and outside the organisation.

The power of metaphors

Section **Two**

COMMUNICATION IN ORGANISATIONS

OVERVIEW

This section of the book focuses on communication skills which impact on the organisation and on ways to influence how an organisation operates. The first four chapters centred on things the reader can do to develop their individual skills. The next three chapters, while incorporating aspects of personal skill, impact beyond the immediate one-to-one situation or the need to influence another person. In these chapters the emphasis is more on how skills can be developed to reach larger numbers of people.

In Chapter Five on communicating in groups, the author provides insight into the ways in which groups act and how knowledge of this can assist effective communication in such settings. In the clinical world the most common group scenario for many nurses will be the clinical team. While many might argue that such groups do not always act as true teams, they provide a useful commonly experienced situation against which the points made in the chapter can be set to assist better understanding. In the world of health service management a good understanding of how groups work and the roles participants assume in meetings, workshops and other interprofessional settings will enable the individual to know what is going on and how group dynamics might prevent or encourage the achievement of positive outcomes.

Presentation to groups has been a required skill for nurses, whether they are clinically or managerially focused, for many years. Whether they present well is more open to question. It is unlikely that most nurses will be natural presenters and there seems to be little emphasis in pre-registration programmes on developing these skills. However, the majority of nurses are likely at some point in their career to need to learn how to present to and engage an audience. Chapter Six on presentation to groups provides a wealth of practical advice on how to master required equipment, maintain the attention of an audience and get across the key issues on what might be a complex subject.

Finally, a chapter on networking is included. This acknowledges the growing importance of developing professional networks as an aid to creating greater awareness of issues and the role of the nurse manager in developing them. Networking allows the non-nursing fraternity to understand issues that they might not appreciate easily without assistance from the right person. There is a growing need to establish nursing and non-medical clinical issues in the complex arena of health service politics if this crucial aspect of the work of NHS organisations is not to be lost. In addition to this, networking allows the individual to become better known in their peer group and beyond. Such a consideration is not necessarily vain as it is becoming increasingly clear that a good network is essential to the career aspirations of the well-motivated, skilled and capable nurse or clinical professional.

All chapters include a variety of applications to illustrate key themes or points made in the main text.

Chapter **Five**

Communication in groups

Linda Ewles

- ● **Types of groups**
- ● **Understanding groups**
- ● **Participating effectively in meetings**
- ● **Managing meetings and leading groups**
- ● **Core skills of communicating in groups**
- ● **Working in groups with other agencies**

O V E R V I E W

Whether you work in hospital, primary care or community, as a manager or the most junior member of staff, you will often find that you are a member of a group or a team. Being able to work and communicate effectively in a group is an important skill for all clinicians because you will need to participate in, or lead, formal and informal group meetings with colleagues and patients. The advent of managed care, protocols and clinical guidelines and the need for wider and wider groups of professionals to communicate about these mean that the team rather than the professional group will increasingly become the main locus of care.

In this chapter, the author aims to identify the range of groups a clinical manager is likely to work with. Key principles are outlined that will help clinicians to ensure that groups work effectively. Group behaviour is discussed along with participation and leadership and related practical skills the clinical manager will find helpful in group or team communication.

93

Finally an overview of how to benefit from attending meetings is included. Indeed many of the issues discussed throughout the chapter are applicable to meetings which are, of course, a particular kind of group experience. As the demands on clinical managers rise in the modern heath service, the ability to function in meetings is becoming ever more important. Indeed, many clinical professionals complain that there are too many meetings but they are likely to remain an important medium for communicating, negotiating and making decisions. So all members of the clinical team need to understand how to get the most benefit from meetings and to feel comfortable in them. Failure to do this will have a negative impact on colleagues, available resources and ultimately on patient care. The key is to learn how to maximise the benefit of meetings so that time away from the clinical area is well spent.

TYPES OF GROUPS

Groups are not random collections of individuals; group members have a sense of shared identity, common objectives, defined membership criteria and their own particular ways of working.

Groups are formed for a variety of purposes. For nurses and other clinical groups, they can be broadly divided into two categories:

- groups of health workers and colleagues, perhaps as a team working together on a ward or in a GP practice. These groups or teams may include a range of professionals such as doctors, therapists, nurses and social workers
- groups of clients, patients or carers, for example a rehabilitation group for patients recovering from heart attacks or a group about parenting skills for new parents.

The context may vary widely and your fellow group members may be very diverse but the core principles and skills we discuss in this chapter can be applied to any kind of group.

UNDERSTANDING GROUPS

Basic principles

There are two key principles that are important to ensure effective communication and working relationships between people in groups.

- *Respect people as partners* – treat other people in the group as partners, recognising and building on their strengths, developing their self-confidence and mutual trust.
- *Listen* – actively listen to the other people in the group, so that you clearly understand their opinions, thoughts and feelings.

These may seem obvious, commonsense principles until you consider how often you may have been in a group where they were not heeded; where, for example, there was mistrust or lack of appreciation of what people could contribute, people's views overridden without adequate consideration, domination by a few people or by the group leader or most senior person. Any of these factors can leave you wondering why you bothered to attend.

Working in a team

A group all clinical staff will experience is the clinical or multiprofessional team, consisting of nurses, other health professionals and perhaps people from disciplines outside the health service such as social work. Successful teams tend to have the following characteristics.

- A common purpose and shared objectives which are known and agreed by all members.
- Members selected because they have relevant expertise.
- Members who know and agree their own role and know the roles of the other members.
- Members who support each other in achieving the common purpose.
- Members who trust each other and communicate in an open, honest way.
- A leader whose authority is accepted by all members.

Teams also tend to work well together if people play specific roles. A classic study of the characteristics of members of groups by Belbin (1981) concluded that a mix of eight roles is needed for fully effective groups.

- *The Leader* – coordinates the efforts of the group and enables it to work effectively.
- *The Shaper* – is action oriented and encourages the group to get on with its tasks.
- *The Plant* – is the creative source of ideas and proposals.
- *The Monitor/Evaluator* – is good at analysing and criticising.
- *The Resource Investigator* – has a good network of contacts and liaises with other people and agencies.

Communication in groups

● *The Company Worker* – is good at organising and administration.
● *The Team Worker* – supports the members of the group and is a good listener.
● *The Finisher* – contributes foresight and perseverance to ensure that the group completes its tasks.

Each person may play a variety of these roles in a group and most people have their preferred roles. If one or more of these roles is lacking, another member or the team leader can help to make a group more successful by consciously adopting a new role or helping someone else to do so.

Group behaviour

You will be able to work in a group more effectively if you are aware of the ways in which people are likely to behave when they come together in groups (sometimes called 'group dynamics').

Groups tend to show a particular pattern of behaviour as they mature and develop. This developmental cycle has been categorised as having four stages (Tuckman 1965).

Forming

The group is in the process of being established. People meet each other and get to know one another, with individuals establishing their own identity and role within the group. The group's purpose and way of working are established.

Storming

Most groups go through a conflict stage when the leadership and ways in which the group is working are challenged. For example, people may question how things are being done, what the leader's role is and may get into heated discussions with each other. This can be a difficult period for both leader and members but it is a vital stage in the group's maturing process, rather like the period of rebelling and questioning during adolescence. Successful handling of this period leads to the development of open communication, trust and shared responsibility for achieving the purposes of the group.

Norming

At this stage the group settles down, with the norms and accepted practices of the group established.

Performing

The group is fully effective at this stage and is able to concentrate on its tasks.

When the developmental process fails in some way, backstage politicking and attempts to sabotage the group may occur. It is thus worth investing time and effort to help new groups to develop successfully.

Many groups have a limited timespan, meeting for a set number of sessions or until a particular task has been completed. At the end of a group's life, it is natural for members to feel a sense of loss. It may be helpful to spend time in the final session 'rounding up', which could give group members an opportunity to express their appreciation of each other and the completion of their task.

PARTICIPATING EFFECTIVELY IN MEETINGS

Meetings – formal and informal – are one particular kind of group activity. They are notorious for producing heart-sink but a well-run meeting can be enjoyable and productive.

First, here is some guidance on how to be an effective participant at meetings. You may not be in charge but there are a number of constructive things you can do to help a meeting go well.

- Encourage the person chairing the meeting into good practices; for example, ask for clarification on the purpose of the meeting or for a summary of what has been agreed at the end.
- Come prepared, having given some thought to what you would like to get out of the meeting and having read any relevant papers.
- Arrive on time. If you think the meeting is likely to run over time, make a request at the beginning of the meeting for a punctual finish.
- Agree what to do about taking notes: does each person take their own or does one person take them and circulate a copy to everyone else? Do you want detailed notes of everything you discussed or just action points? If it's not clear, ask for clarification and even volunteer to do the notes yourself.
- Do not speak for too long – just a minute or two at a time should be long enough to make your point.
- Actively contribute to the meeting – express your views, keep an open mind and listen to other people's opinions.
- Encourage everyone to participate – draw in quieter people by referring to their relevant experience or expertise.

Communication in groups

- Only make commitments that you are genuinely able to fulfil and make sure you do so on time. Say 'no' clearly and non-defensively if you are unable or unwilling to do something.
- Remember that discussion and argument about ideas will help decision making but personal rivalries will not.

Effective committee work

All health care professionals will increasingly be required to become members of formal committees or boards; for example, there are nurse members of primary health care trusts. This can be daunting if you have never served on a formal committee before and it helps to know the basic rules of how they work.

A committee is a group of people appointed for a specific purpose accountable to a larger group or organisation; examples are the management committee of a voluntary organisation or the health committee of a local authority. The officers are servants of the committee and carry out its instructions. Many committees have three key officers: the chair, the secretary and the treasurer. As committees grow the officers often need help with their work and additional appointments may be necessary; for example, a minutes secretary.

Committees tend to be informal nowadays but it is good to bear in mind the reasons for accepted codes of behaviour. For example, the rule that only one person speaks at a time, and is not interrupted, is meant to ensure a fair hearing for everyone. The rule of everyone speaking by addressing the meeting through the chair helps to prevent a number of sub-discussions developing at the same time. On the other hand, it may seem more natural and helpful to address another committee member directly. Ultimately it is the job of the chair to set the tone which encourages all members to participate whilst keeping the meeting under control.

MANAGING MEETINGS AND LEADING GROUPS

If you are required to lead a group or chair a meeting, it is useful to think about two aspects: your responsibilities as a group leader and your leadership style.

Leadership responsibilities

If you have the task of leading a group or running meetings, your key responsibilities will probably include:

- helping participants to identify and clarify their interests and needs and what they would like to gain from the group or meeting, in the short and long term
- helping to develop a relaxed atmosphere in which people feel able to be open and trusting with each other and able to participate freely
- offering your expertise to the group
- accepting and valuing all contributions from participants.

Leadership style

Not everyone will lead a group in the same way and it is helpful to be aware of your own preferred style of leadership. A key dimension is where you stand on a continuum from authoritarian to participative.

An *authoritarian style* group leader acts as a 'director' who is a source of expertise. If you adopt this approach, you rely on your status, credibility and expertise to ensure acceptance of your views and leadership role. The *strength* of this style is that people who are new to the job or unsure of themselves may feel secure and reassured. The *weakness* is that group members may become dependent on you and reluctant to take independent action. Alternatively, the more strong-minded members may respond by rebelling and rejecting your guidance.

A *participative style* involves shifting power from the group leader so that it is shared between the leader and the group members. This means using all the skills and knowledge of the group members as well as the leader, who will act as more of a facilitator than a leader. The *strength* of this style is that group members learn to trust their own judgements and at the same time to appreciate other people's rights and opinions. The *weakness* is that people who are used to being told what to do may feel confused and dissatisfied because they are not receiving the direction they want. They may need to have the approach explained to them.

A participative style must be distinguished from a *permissive* style where the leader lets group members come to their own conclusions and aims to avoid conflict and keep everyone happy. This rarely works; often goals are not achieved and nobody is satisfied. Difficulties and conflict are not confronted. Group leaders may need to build up their own assertiveness skills in order to avoid an overly permissive approach.

There is no 'right' or 'wrong' style and indeed most leaders probably operate somewhere between the two extremes, providing

Communication in groups

some authoritative leadership while also encouraging a degree of participation.

It is commonly assumed that groups will be more effective with a participative rather than authoritarian leadership style but the reality of leadership is more complex and successful group leadership depends on a variety of factors including the following.

- The leader's preferred style of operating and personality. For example, if you have been used to being perceived as the 'expert' with the authority of professional knowledge which you want to pass on, you will probably feel (and look) uncomfortable if you try to switch to a 'facilitator' style without sufficient training and this will produce tension in the group.
- The group members' preferred style of leadership in the specific circumstances of the group. For example, if group members are low in confidence, they may need you to be more authoritarian to start with, so that they feel secure. You can then gradually encourage participation and adopt a more facilitative style as members learn to trust you and each other and feel confident enough to join in.
- The group's objectives and tasks. For example, a group which has the objective of learning new skills will need a more authoritarian leader to teach them the skills. But a paediatric nurse who is leading a support group for bereaved parents will need a facilitation approach to help people to express and work through their grief.

You need to consider these factors and how they might be modified, in order to achieve the 'best fit'.

Setting ground rules

People joining a group or attending a meeting may have different expectations and assumptions about how it will run. Problems may arise if these are not brought out into the open and clarified at the beginning. For example, people may assume that what they say in a group will be treated confidentially, then be upset if they find that another person did not realise this and has discussed the issue elsewhere. To prevent these difficulties, it is often helpful to establish a clear 'contract' or 'set of ground rules'. So early on in the life of a group members need the opportunity to explore their expectations, and reach agreement, about issues such as the following.

- How people are expected to behave in the group. For example, is it OK to arrive late?

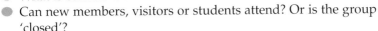

- What is confidential?
- Can new members, visitors or students attend? Or is the group 'closed'?
- How will the leader and the members exercise control in the group?
- Who has responsibility for the practical aspects of running the group, such as setting the agenda or taking notes?

Practical points

The location and seating in the place where you hold your meeting can make a big difference and are worth considering if you have any choice in the matter. A setting such as a board room is likely to result in a formal atmosphere. If you want an informal session with everyone contributing, seating people on easy chairs in a circle is best, with physical barriers to communication such as tables or desks removed. Cups of tea and coffee help to relax people and bis-cuits or sandwiches always help if busy people have not had time to eat.

CORE SKILLS OF COMMUNICATING IN GROUPS

Getting groups going

Almost everyone feels nervous about going to a group meeting for the first time, especially if they do not know anyone else there. The initial task for a group leader is to 'break the ice' and help people to feel at ease.

On arrival

It helps if people can be greeted personally and introduced to other people. Giving people something to do also helps: 'Help yourself to a cup of tea'. Ensure that anyone with special needs has appro-priate facilities and assistance (e.g. with mobility or hearing loops).

Getting to know each other

Knowing each person's name and something about them helps people to feel that everyone is a valued member of the group; this is the beginning of openness and trust between members. If, for

Communication in groups

example, a team is meeting for the first time, the simplest way is just to ask people to say their name, their job, a perhaps a word or two about their background and experience. It helps if the group leader or chair sets the tone by going first.

If the group you are leading has a different aim, you may like to break the ice more thoroughly. For example, if you are a midwife running a group for prospective parents, you could ask people to sit next to someone they have not met before and chat to that person. Perhaps asking specific questions would help such as: is this is your first baby, where are you going for antenatal check-ups, where are you booked to have your baby? After a few minutes (the leader keeps the time) the partners swap roles and the other person is interviewed. Then, in turn, members of the group introduce their partner by name and say something about them. You may like to remind people that no-one has to answer any questions if they do not wish to.

At subsequent group meetings, it is often helpful to do a quick round of names at the beginning, e.g. 'Who would like to have a shot at naming every member of the group?' or 'I'm going to see if I can remember everyone's name'.

Discussion skills

It is a fallacy to believe that leading a discussion will just happen by putting a group of people together and saying 'Let's discuss . . .'. Discussion needs planning and preparation and there are many ways of triggering it off and providing structures which will help everyone to participate. Some of these are as follows.

Trigger materials

Discussion can be triggered by providing a focus, preferably a controversial one. This can simply be a question ('What do you think about the proposal to change the way we deal with emergency admissions?') or it might be a leaflet, a poster, a video or an item in a newspaper or magazine. (For example, in a smoking cessation group 'What do you think the makers of this cigarette are trying to convey in this advertisement?'.) Choose something that people are likely to have strong views about.

Brainstorming

This is a useful way to open up a subject and collect everyone's ideas. Ask an open question to which there is no single right answer ('Why are we not meeting our targets?'). Accept every suggestion, without comment or criticism, and write them down in a list on a flipchart or whiteboard. Alternatively, write each idea separately on a sticky note (the kind you can peel off and move) and put these on a flipchart. Ask the group not to start discussing the ideas until everybody has finished. You can make your own suggestions and write them down along with everyone else's.

In this way all members' contributions are equally valued and everyone has a chance to participate. Encourage shy members by asking 'Anything else?' and allowing silent pauses while people think.

Then you can set the group to work by asking them to put the ideas into categories and to identify the key features of each category.

Rounds

A 'round' is a way of giving everyone an equal chance to participate. You invite each person in turn to make a brief statement. You may like to start the round yourself or to join in when your turn comes. For example, ask everyone to make a brief statement about one of the following:

● 'The thing which stresses me most is . . . '
● 'The thing I think would help most with this problem is . . . '

There are four essential rules for successful rounds, which should be explained and gently enforced if necessary. These are:

● no interruptions until each person has finished their statement
● no comments on anybody's contribution until the full round is completed (i.e. no discussions, praise, interpretation, criticism or I-think-that-too type of remark)
● anyone can choose not to participate. Give permission, clearly and emphatically, that anyone who does not want to make a statement can just say 'pass'
● it does not matter if two or more people in the round say the same thing. People should stick to saying what they had intended to say even if someone else has said it already; they do not have to think of something different.

Rounds are also useful ways of beginning and ending sessions. For example:

● 'One thing I've put into practice since last week is . . . '
● 'The main thing I've got from today's session is . . . '
● 'One thing I'm going to find out by next time we meet is . . . '

Communication in groups

It is also a useful way of getting feedback. For example:

- 'One thing I really liked about today's meeting was . . . '
- 'One thing I wish we'd done is . . . '

Dealing with difficulties

People often find the prospect of leading a group or managing a meeting quite daunting and anticipate being unable to cope with problems. A way forward is to acknowledge and face these fears and work out strategies for coping should the problem actually arise. Some common fears and possible strategies are as follows.

Silence

Are you afraid that you may be left with your group in an awful silence? If so, remember that silence can be useful; it can be time which group members need for thinking. Silence often does not feel as threatening to group members as it does to you. However, you may find it helpful to:

- run a group with a colleague, so that you can help each other out if either of you gets stuck
- ensure thorough preparation, so that you have a planned agenda for a meeting or a set of activities and questions for a group to work on. Write down your agenda or plan and don't be afraid to refer to it in front of the group
- have a 'spare' activity ready to use if what you have planned does not seem to be working.

Disasters

Unexpected 'disasters' include such things as getting lost and arriving late or finding that too few or too many people have turned up. There is no blueprint strategy to cope with the unexpected but it will help if you acknowledge what has happened and share it with your group ('I'm delighted that so many of you have come along, but I wasn't expecting such a crowd, so we may be a bit squashed this week'). Also share your plans for dealing with the 'disaster' ('I'm going to try to get a bigger room next time' . . . 'I'm going to start 10 minutes late'). Sharing the problem and enlisting cooperation can have the positive benefit of encouraging mutual support; *not* sharing it can leave your group feeling angry.

Distractions

Distractions can take many forms: noises outside the room (e.g. road works), noises inside the room (e.g. crying babies, coughing), people coming in late or leaving early, or interruptions. Group members can also cause distractions themselves, for example by becoming angry or upset.

As a rule, there are three choices for you as group leader.

● Ignore the problem. This is seldom a good idea, as it leaves people wondering whether you are going to do anything and this in itself is a distraction.

● Acknowledge and accept it. This is generally best with things you cannot change ('I know the traffic is really noisy, but there's nothing we can do about it, so I think we'll just have to put up with it').

● Do something about it. It is preferable to involve the group in the decision ('As so many of you found it difficult to get here by 2 pm, shall we start at 2.15 next week?').

If someone is showing emotion, such as crying, acknowledge it ('I can see that you're upset'), offer reassurance that it is OK to show emotion ('There's no need to be embarrassed . . . we don't mind if you cry . . . ') and offer the opportunity to talk about it ('Would you like to tell us what is upsetting you?') or to take some time away from the group, accompanied by you or someone else ('Shall we go outside for a few minutes?'). Do not put any pressure on people in distress. Help them to do what they want to do, whether it is crying, talking, keeping silent, staying, leaving or being by themselves. But do not ignore a show of emotion; ignoring it will only cause tension and embarrassment.

Difficult behaviour

People's behaviour can pose difficulties for a group leader or the chair of a meeting. There are two broad categories of difficult behaviour: non-participation and talking too much. The latter category takes many forms, such as the know-all who always chips in with all the 'answers' and people who launch into long stories, interrupt, do not let other people get a word in edgeways, talk off the point, always disagree or always crack jokes.

Some ways of tackling difficult behaviour are as follows.

● A starting point is to try to think *why* people behave like this. Are they nervous, threatened, worried? Are they desperately in need of attention? If you can deal with the underlying cause, the situation is likely to improve.

- Note that people often change their behaviour as they get to know others and feel more comfortable in a group.
- Try getting people to work in pairs or small groups, which can help quiet members to join in and give others a break from the constant talker.
- Use structures in your discussion, such as 'rounds', or make a point of asking for other people's opinions ('Would someone else like to say what he thinks?', 'Would you like to give us your opinion, Ann?').
- It may be necessary to confront the difficult person (not in front of the rest of the group!). For example, you could say: 'I've noticed that you contribute a great deal to our discussions. That makes me concerned about whether other people are getting enough chance to talk. I'd like to suggest that you keep your comments to just a couple of sentences. Would you feel OK about doing that?'.

Hidden agendas

People will have their own individual reasons for joining a group or for behaving the way they do in a meeting. This may be in addition to, or instead of, the reason expected. For example, someone may seek a dominant position in a group primarily to fulfil a need to be valued and useful; another may be obstructive because of a grudge against the chair. This personal objective is a 'hidden agenda'.

Groups will work together best when there is communication about individual objectives and agreement about shared objectives. Otherwise people may promote their own interests at the expense of the group's. You will be more effective as a group leader if you are aware of the hidden agendas in the group and can find ways of dealing with them.

WORKING IN GROUPS WITH OTHER AGENCIES

Increasingly, health care professionals will be working in groups with people not just from other disciplines, but from other agencies. So, for example, a community nurse dealing with child abuse may work with police and social workers. Multiagency groups are often called 'partnerships'. The main reasons for setting up a partnership are:

- to harness a range of complementary skills and resources to work towards common goals

- to avoid duplication and fragmentation of effort
- to avoid gaps in services.

Factors for success

Successful health partnerships do not 'just happen': they are usually the result of investing a considerable amount of resources, skill and time in order for members to work well together. Key factors for success are as follows.

- All partners need to be working towards a shared vision of what the partnership should achieve, with an agenda and goals which all partners agree to.
- All partners need to feel a sense of ownership of the partnership and not that one partner dominates, with others as 'second-class' members.
- Commitment from the highest level of member organisations is vital to ensure that group objectives fit with the organisation's strategic aims and that there will be management support for input of time and other resources.
- There must be commitment of sufficient time and resources and realistic expectations; partnership working is time consuming and it may take months or years to develop a shared understanding and joint plans, let alone achieve results from joint activities. On the other hand, there must be demonstrable achievements, otherwise the partnership will be regarded as a mere 'talking shop'.
- Someone acceptable to all partners needs to take responsibility for running the partnership (for example, setting up, chairing and servicing meetings) and coordinating action.
- There must be mutual respect between partners; all partners need to feel that others value their input.
- Working relationships need to be characterised by openness and trust.
- There needs to be an agreed framework for reviewing the partnership, changing the way of working, if necessary, and even bringing it to an end if the partnership has outlived its usefulness or is unproductive.

Potential difficulties

Partnerships can face many difficulties. Major problems are:

- organisational change, which blights long-term commitment and planning

107

- professional jealousy and unwillingness to share expertise and information
- lack of resources, both money and person-power
- lack of top-level commitment from agencies on the partnership
- individual personalities who dominate a partnership
- an imbalance of input from different agencies which can lead to resentment, issues of ownership of joint activities and who takes the credit for success
- differences between agencies and individuals in terms of different goals and values, different organisational cultures and ways of working, different levels of expertise and experience.

It is worth bearing in mind that not all partnerships are successful. Many may fade out or be wound up. Partnerships are not an end in themselves, they are a means to an end, and there may be circumstances where the end is better achieved by an organisation working alone.

CONCLUSION

All health care professionals need to work in groups, respecting other members as partners, listening to their views and understanding their feelings. Working teams can be built up with knowledge of the factors important for success and an understanding of group behaviour. Practising skills of helpful participation in meetings will contribute to effective outcomes rather than heart-sink and if you have responsibility for leading groups or meetings, you need to know what your responsibilities are, adopt the appropriate leadership style, pay attention to ground rules and practical points such as seating arrangements. Core skills of group work are vital, including how to get groups going, trigger discussion and deal with difficulties and hidden agendas. Multiagency partnership working poses other challenges but an understanding of key factors for success and potential difficulties can help to make these partnerships more effective.

> ### Practice checklist
>
> As a means of developing more effective group communication skills you may find it helpful to use a checklist such as the one below. It is important to remember that such lists only provide a framework of the areas of knowledge and skill you need to develop. You need to understand the basic principles which

Communication in organisations

Practice checklist (*Cont.*)

underpin effective group communication and teamwork and the way in which groups usually develop over time.

- For effective meetings and committee work, you require knowledge of how people behave in meetings, the roles and responsibilities of members and skills of making the most of meetings and committees.
- If you run groups or meetings, you will find it helpful to think about your leadership responsibilities and style, setting ground rules and other practical points.
- You will need core skills of communicating in groups, including how to get groups going, encourage discussion and deal with difficulties.
- Groups often involve different professionals and disciplines working together in partnerships; there is a range of ways in which you can encourage good teamwork and coordination.

Discussion questions

- Make a list of all the groups you belong to: work teams, working groups, project groups, committees, task groups, professional associations. Discuss whether they work well or not: rank them on a scale of 1 to 5: 1 = works very well, 5 = works very badly. What criteria have you used to say that a group works 'well' or not? What are the reasons for working well? What factors contribute to poor group work?
- Select one or two groups you belong to and think about whether you could take steps to make the group function better. The principles outlined in this chapter could give you the necessary conceptual framework to guide you.
- Identify three or four ways in which you could develop your skills of communication in groups and set yourself an action plan.

Having answered these questions you will begin to see some of the features described in the groups you participate in or at the meetings you attend. As with most things, practice is important and it will be of value to repeat the exercises above with new groups you join until you are sufficiently familiar with the tools and technique to do it automatically.

Communication in groups

Acknowledgement

We acknowledge, with thanks, that much of the material in this chapter is adapted from Ewles L, Simnett I 1999 Promoting health – a practical guide, 4th edn. Baillière Tindall, London

References

Belbin RM 1981 Management teams: why they succeed or fail. Butterworth Heinemann, Oxford

Tuckman BW 1965 Developmental sequence in small groups. Psychological Bulletin 63: 384–399

Further reading

Belbin M 1996 Management teams – why they succeed or fail. Butterworth, London

Belbin M 1996 Team roles at work. Butterworth, London

Benne K, Sheats P 1948 Functional roles of group members. Journal of Social Issues 4: 41–49

Berne E 1968 Games people play. Penguin, Harmondsworth

Bormann EG, Bormann NC 1988 Effective small group communication, 4th edn. Burgess, Edina, Minnesota

Ewles L, Simnett I 1999 Promoting health – a practical guide, 4th edn. Baillière Tindall, London

Hartley P 1997 Group communication. Routledge, London

Margerison C, McCann D 1985 How to lead a winning team. MCB University Press, Bradford

Steiner ID 1972 Group processes and productivity. Academic Press, New York

Tubbs S 1995 A systems approach to small group interaction. McGraw-Hill, New York

How presentation to a meeting can promote clinical work

INTRODUCTION

At an acute Trust the Director of Nursing became aware of excellent work to implement integrated care pathways (ICPs) on the cardiology unit. The unit charge nurse had worked with the medical staff and colleagues from the allied health professions to agree the principles for establishing ICPs to improve quality in patient care. The main outcome was documentation that was enthusiastically received by all clinical staff and that was well used by patients. The problem was that this excellent work was limited to the one unit with no apparent signs that other clinical areas were willing to adopt this approach to care. With the advent of clinical governance it was important to continually improve clinical quality and ICPs were a way to do this.

The Director of Nursing was aware of the need to extend this work throughout the Trust, which required the support of the Trust Board. The Director was aware that it was never easy to present a primarily nursing-led initiative to non-clinical staff. It was agreed that the coronary care unit staff should attend a Board meeting and present the outcomes of their work at a clinical update session.

THE BOARD MEETING

Although this seemed a relatively straightforward meeting a number of factors had to be considered if success was to be assured. The Board was a mixture of clinical and non-clinical directors and senior managers who worked alongside five non-executive directors, none of whom had a clinical background. The presentation to the meeting would therefore need to be intelligible to a range of people. It was decided to adopt an approach that set out the aims and objectives of the work along with key clinical factors in a clear manner that avoided where possible the use of 'jargon' or professionally understood acronyms to allow all to understand the presentation.

Issues relating to who would present, what style of audiovisual support would be used and whether staff would wear uniforms or not were discussed. Handouts were designed and examples of the unit documentation were prepared. Staff who would be presenting visited the Trust boardroom prior to the event to familiarise themselves with the layout of the room.

The Director of Nursing gained the support of the Medical Director by informing him of the potential importance of this work to their joint activities on clinical governance. He in turn assured himself that the unit Clinical Director (who was to be present) was fully supportive of the work to date. The Chief Executive and the Trust Chairwoman were also briefed. Finally, the presence of the Director of Nursing – though not integral to the presentation – would ensure that any difficult moments in the meeting could be handled.

One key aspect of the meeting was the decision to focus on informing the non-executive directors. By engaging their support, an important precedent in Trust business was achieved wherein requests for more examples be put to the Board in future.

The presentation and subsequent discussion at the meeting was a great success. More regular clinical updates were planned to feature nursing innovation; traditionally the sessions had been reserved for medical work. This showed that a thorough and professional approach to an important presentation to a key group in the Trust not only gained the planned outcome but resulted in an unexpected one too.

Throughout the meeting the key principles of good presentation were employed including: speaking clearly and at the right pace, knowing your audience, avoiding confusing or obscure language, use of well-prepared audiovisual aids, awareness of the strengths and limitations of the venue and preparedness for questions. Not only was board level support forthcoming but presenting the initiative guaranteed senior management support for using the approach to achieve clinical governance. In addition, hitherto unknown staff gained recognition for their work which led to agreement on a secondment to promote, support and coordinate this work.

Chapter **Six**

Presentations to groups

Brenda Maslen

- **Core issues**
- **Audiovisual aids**
- **Capturing the audience's attention**
- **Keeping the material interesting**
- **Management of self**
- **Interactions with the media**

Presentations to groups

O V E R V I E W

This chapter examines and discusses the issues associated with giving presentations to groups of people from a number of perspectives. Increasingly members of all health care professions are being required to justify the case for resources or staff in a management environment. Also, new ideas on practice are developing at a rapid pace. Both of these developments will at some point require the clinical professional to make some sort of presentation either to colleagues at clinical level or those in management.

The author covers purely functional aspects of presentation as well as ideas and concepts related to how the individual manages their preparation to give an efficient and effective performance. These two major aspects are dependent one upon the other. If the experience is also enjoyable, which it is hoped will be encouraged by using the advice in this chapter, this is an added bonus. This major and growing aspect of communication at work must be understood and mastered if success is to be more certain when competing for resources, conveying new ideas or attempting to change or influence practice.

113

INTRODUCTION

A manager's job is said to be as much about communication as anything else (Stewart 1992). Whilst listening is also as much a part of this as talking, those in a management role need to be able to get the message across to subordinates, peers, senior managers and indeed anyone with whom meaningful interaction is sought. Giving presentations with a high level of skill has therefore become an intrinsic part of the working environment. One way of working proactively is to sell your ideas to your boss and upper management, the key prerequisite of this process being that what you are selling is something they need or will at least benefit from. This could be called a 'win-win' proposition. In addition to enhancing your own organisational power, it is important to actively empower the people who work with or for you.

Health care is no exception to this general ethos and, amongst other things, presentations offer a useful method of selling an idea, reporting back on courses or conferences attended, publishing innovations in your working environment, teaching staff and clients and literally selling yourself as part of the interview process. Knowledge and skills in this field put you in a position to comment and contribute in an informed manner to events which you attend and cascade information in the organisation, maximising the value-for-money ethos which is prevalent in today's health care facilities.

The simplest use of presentation as a technique is to give information and the list of topics is endless. A decision must be taken as to the topic and the purpose. Although you will have an agenda to pursue as the initiator of the process it is important to ensure that the needs of the target audience are met.

Many of the other chapters in this book are complementary to what you will learn from this one and are equally applicable to all professional groups. Similarly, theory offered here can be applied to other situations. As the material offered is generic in nature, it will be important for you to apply it to your own particular needs. Suggestions will be given as to how you might achieve this.

No book or written publication can replace the experience of practical activity and taking the maxim that you learn from what you actually do – rather than from what you see and hear – having the courage to try out your own ideas will be the lynchpin of your personal success. You may need to stop thinking about it and just do it! Waiting until you think you can do it perfectly may be the difference between proaction and inaction.

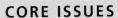

CORE ISSUES

Whatever the purpose of the presentation there are core issues which impact upon the success of what occurs. Developing a deeper understanding of these will enable you to be more effective in achieving your goals.

Physical comfort

Dependent upon the purpose of the activity, seating should be arranged in order to enhance what occurs. Therefore, if it is going to be vital for people to be able to see each other's faces then a horseshoe shape or circle may be appropriate. If, however, as in a standard lecture theatre, the audience is large and the focus of attention is to be on the speaker then tiers of seats are not only acceptable but probably essential.

If you have control over the environment in which the presentation is to occur it will be important to ensure that the audience will be comfortable. This includes such things as seating, lighting, heating, safety issues and the acoustics and visibility range of the venue. This may seem a foregone conclusion but if you have ever had to sit through a presentation with chattering teeth or perspiring freely you will know that the one message that remains after the event is the discomfort you felt. Of course, if you are a visiting speaker you will not have the same control over these factors and it might be worth checking out these kinds of issues prior to the actual event as it can be difficult once you begin your presentation. You could perhaps utilise the checklist in Application 6.1 to do this.

Language, including paralanguage

At a macro level awareness of English or other languages employed by the group is fundamental to the success of the venture. However, there are many other linguistic anomalies which include such matters as professional terms or elaborated codes which are more obscure and it is therefore important that you assess the audience before deciding on the type of language to use.

There is a general awareness of antidiscriminatory legislation which vetoes any inappropriate comments. However, general usage, custom, habit and upbringing may all contribute to errors being made and it is therefore essential, without spoiling the sense and rhythm of what you want to say or being overcensorious, that you try to avoid insulting anyone in your audience.

Paralanguage is the non-verbal aspect of speech. There are a number of tools for making your voice more interesting such as volume, pitch and inflection, pace and rhythm. Emphasis affects your word and syllable stress and the key here is to be sure people get your main ideas. In addition to this, your attitude can make the same words take on radically different meanings. An example of this might be when you have planned a picnic and it is a fine sunny day. The way you say 'Isn't this a lovely day for a picnic?' would vary greatly from the way in which you would say it if it was pouring down with rain!

Remember that anxiety is likely to raise the pitch of your voice by about one tone. What people see and hear fundamentally influence the message you wish to transmit and image you wish to portray.

Management of information

Any information presented must make sense and, more importantly, it must make sense to those who are receiving it. When you design a presentation its success will depend upon the logical progression of information at a pace and in a format which will appeal to the audience. They must be able to identify links to previous knowledge and in this way understand what is being discussed. Thus you proceed from the known to the unknown.

In this context, making the meaning clear can be supported by using an oral or written headline. Just as in the newspapers where a headline tells the reader what the following story is all about, you can give the audience a good idea of how to make sense of what follows.

Take care with the amount and type of material to be used or presented. Having too much material is a stress-reducing strategy often used by those who are not used to speaking to a group. Although silence itself is an important communication strategy, newcomers to the stage often fear an uncomfortable silence but the outcome of having prepared a large amount of material can be a feeling of pressure to get it all delivered. In this process the core message may get lost, leaving the audience completely bewildered.

Whilst observing trainee teachers, it is evident that they often prepare too much material and are unwilling to let any of it go. This results in hasty or non-existent endings and endings are as important as beginnings.

With regard to the type of material to use, Boisot (1987, cited in Stewart 1992) developed a method of classifying information conveyed to others in two dimensions.

- Can it be coded easily (where one end of the continuum is highly structured and can be symbolically represented, e.g. by figures, and the other is vague and full of intangible ideas)?
- Can it be easily disseminated (by what means and relevantly to an appropriate audience)?

If motivation is taken as an example, in trying to motivate an individual a large lecture may give some intellectual insights but will probably do little to motivate. One-to-one discussion would be far better. By contrast, sales figures are easily identifiable, will be widely understood and thus can be conveyed in writing or even in a lecture with slides.

The recipients of the information need an opportunity to ask questions. This can be managed by offering to accept questions throughout the presentation, which can sometimes be risky regarding control of material and timing, or by allowing a specific period for this at the end of the presentation. This has its own dangers and can result in an uncomfortable silence occurring.

If you wish group members to feel that they have come to a conclusion themselves then Socratic questioning may be used (Walklin 1990). This method, as its name suggests, was refined by Socrates, using a series of carefully planned questions which lead the audience in a step-by-step fashion to some statement of principle, solution of a problem or a conclusion. It may be seen as much more valuable than a closed questioning technique as it does not rely purely on fact or memory but on reasoning, speculation and extended use of knowledge.

Appearance

Lasting opinions are formed from first impressions and, dependent upon the occasion, you will need to dress and conduct yourself according to the image you wish to portray. However, an element of authenticity is important as those with whom you are trying to establish contact can often see through an assumed image, however well it is portrayed. This applies equally to appearance, verbal and non-verbal behaviour.

In order to address these core skills use the following checklist.

- Preparation of material – relevence, amount, sequence.
- Appearance – what image do I want to portray?

- Comfort – temperature, lighting, heating, seating, safety.
- Speech – clarity, volume, pitch, content, discriminatory remarks.

It might also help to consider the following.

- What is the purpose of this presentation?
- Who are the audience?
- What are their needs?
- What time do I have available?
- What am I going to include?
- How am I going to measure my success?

This last point is essential with regard to personal reflection as part of your own learning cycle but you will not always be able to seek feedback from the audience. However, if it is appropriate, the opinions of others can be invaluable to developing your technique and you may wish to offer the audience a feedback form to complete.

Presentation technique

The technique for giving a good presentation is to remember that most people are only able to concentrate for relatively short periods of time. Changes in timing, providing spaces or pauses and leading activities or questions should be incorporated into the presentation to take account of this.

Many experienced after-dinner speakers would advocate starting with something which quickly engages the attention of the audience. Once you have gained their attention, do not disappoint them – they will have expectations of you and these must sit comfortably with you as a person. It is important, therefore, that your opening gambit is not something borrowed from someone else whose agenda you would be unable to follow. It is generally accepted that the use of illustrations of one sort or another enhances a presentation and this will be discussed later on in this chapter.

If you incorporate the core skills checklist into your work you will already be on the way to success but it is in the technique that the maxim 'It's not what you say, it's the way that you say it' will very much come into play. You can have very good material, a wonderful idea, a meaningful suggestion but if you do not present it appropriately all can be lost. This does not mean that you need to be an 'all-singing, all-dancing failed entertainer' to make an impact, for not everyone can carry this off, but it does mean that you must show enthusiasm when trying to sell an idea. How you do this will be down to your personality but if you are quiet then you will need to show enthusiasm quietly!!

Sanders (1992) quotes Lord Curzon (1859–1925) who was recognised as a fine orator and who made the following perceptive statement about audiences. He said the three most important things to remember are:

- who you are – your personality, relevant knowledge and experience. You must engage the whole of your physical self – voice, eyes, face, hands, arms – to assist communication. Don't completely overwhelm the audience but don't be overmodest either. Anecdotes often stick in the mind
- how you say it – the best use of your voice. Every effort should be made to increase and enlarge the vocal range and to keep the voice in trim with constant exercising
- what you say – requires careful selection and ordering. Everything must be relevant to the particular occasion.

A presentation should have a beginning, a middle and an end and it is important to let your audience know which part you are currently dealing with. Logically section the presentation and keep the audience abreast, by way of short intertalk summaries, charts or direct statements, of the point in the presentation which you have reached.

This could be likened to painting in the background which is a strategy employed by storytellers and scriptwriters, so when you are setting up your story think about what is already inside the other person's mind. Ask yourself 'What can I safely assume they already know?', 'Do they understand the situation I want to talk about?'. The aim is to describe enough of the picture for the other person to begin to 'be there' with you. Be careful to avoid starting your story part way through. For instance, if you've been mulling over something for a while before you talk about it, there is often a temptation to begin the story at the point where you left it in your mind.

Non-verbal elements of your own and the audience's behaviour are important landmarks as to how you are putting over the presentation and how it is being received. A positive stance which is neither overtense (bent backwards) or overpassive (slumped forward) is crucial to your presence on the platform. Gestures are useful, especially when they indicate that you would like the audience to join in with you, but take care with repeated and often unconscious movements, which are known as mannerisms. They can provide a source of amusement to the listener and a source of material to the mimic.

Presentations to groups

The audience's facial expression will alert you as to how they are receiving the material. Glazed or downcast eyes indicate boredom or lack of interest, as does fidgeting. A body position indicating interest is upright, slightly leaning forward and maintaining good eye contact. Fully raised eyebrows indicate disbelief and half-raised eyebrows puzzlement.

AUDIOVISUAL AIDS

Walklin (1990) suggests that to discover for yourself the value of visual aids, you try to describe to a group of people a picture of something that they have never seen or heard of and without showing them the picture. Ask the group to name the 'something' and you will probably receive a wide variety of suggestions.

Most presentations benefit from the use of audiovisual aids and it is likely that these will be prepared beforehand rather than 'live' during the presentation. The systems for producing these can be very simple, for example a hand-drawn chart or acetate, or much more complex, such as a computer-generated image. The type of topic, purpose and group numbers will influence which aid is chosen and the following comprehensive list may prompt ideas.

- Chalkboard
- Marker board
- Flipchart
- Models
- Charts
- Posters
- Real items (equipment)
- Overhead projector
- Films
- Slides
- CCTV
- Video
- Television
- Discs (either music or computer)
- Tapes (audio or video)

It is not possible to describe all of these in detail here but the following are the most likely to be employed.

- *Flipchart* – cheap, advance preparation, illustration or text. Needs artistic ability, legibility, relatively inflexible. Use different coloured pens for emphasis or differentiation. Produce outline, leaving space for additions during the session.

- *Acetate (OHP transparency)* – has the same benefits as flipchart and material can be enlarged by using overhead projector. Useful for small groups and low key meetings. Usually A4 in size and can be horizontal (landscape) or vertical (portrait). If using a word processor or computer, text size 18 is about right or larger if you wish to use key words for impact.
- *35 mm slides* – perhaps for the more important meeting. Need to be prepared by an expert technician or, if preparing yourself, keep text to a minimum, just headings and main points. About six lines of text with 10 words per line would be a useful guide-line. In general terms light lettering on dark backgrounds works best and customising a presentation with a particular slide style can be effective, especially if relevant to the topic. A slide carousel needs expertise for smooth operation. It is usually a good idea to familiarise yourself with available audiovisual support before starting.
- Slides may also be generated with a computer software package such as Microsoft PowerPoint but it is important to remember that computer-generated material needs compatible equipment in order to access it and this may not be available at every venue. However, it can be extremely effective if used well but take care that the technology does not outwit the presenter. I recently saw a presentation where timed changes had been programmed in but the presenter did not keep up with the computer and, worse still, did not check the screen for what it was showing. The result was quite distracting. Just like all methods, practice is essential and, what is more, practice in private rather than with an audience unless of course it is an audience selected for the purpose of assessing the effectiveness of a particular method.
- Video film is notoriously difficult to make and edit but that might be the only way of getting exactly what you want. Professionally produced material can be incorporated into the presentation, but take care with copyright issues.

All these methods allow you to face the audience but always check that you are actually displaying what you intend.

To use these resources effectively once you have prepared them, you should:

- become familiar with them
- check them beforehand for their suitability for the audience and topic
- check any equipment before the presentation to see that it works

121

- check any equipment for safety
- plan for the aids to be shown at the correct time (on some computer-generated material the time lapse can be programmed in to function automatically)
- be able to explain them clearly.

The rationale for using visual material is that it creates an opportunity to focus the minds of the audience on what is being presented, can reinforce a point, introduce diagrammatic material, give you a focus and, by using art or cartoons, can lighten up difficult material.

When preparing aids remember that information displayed should be kept to a minimum. Providing illustrations of highly complex diagrams or tables will detract from your purpose as people just will not read them. Headings, key words, simple flow charts are best.

Although visual aids can enhance a presentation, improper use of them can detract from it. Do not use visual aids simply because it is the done thing; as with your other material, there must be a purpose and meaning. Always check out items you intend to use by looking at them from a distance yourself and inviting comments from others. If using computer-generated material it is sometimes tempting to use all the functions simply because they exist.

CAPTURING THE AUDIENCE'S ATTENTION

Strategies have been mentioned to maintain the attention of the audience but to do this you must first of all attract it. People often end up at presentations if not by accident, then by someone else's design and in order to capture their interest you must start off with something short, interesting, punchy and possibly funny. Although your purpose may not be that of entertainment, you may be able to borrow some ideas from stand-up comedians who know that if you do not capture the audience in the first 30 seconds you have lost them forever. Left to our own devices, our attention turns inward and in effect we hold a conversation with ourselves by listening to our own thoughts. It can take quite an effort to redirect this attention towards someone else, especially if we already have some important things on our mind.

Many speakers agree that making an audience respond positively within the first few minutes is hard work but it must not look like that. One ploy used when presenting information on communication, for example, is to begin the presentation by speaking in a

Communication in organisations

'foreign' language. To further make the point, the author has used a language devised as a child which involves adding the letters 'aga' after every vowel of a word so that there is enough of the familiar for it to sound tantalisingly recognisable, but not quite. You can see the puzzled looks and intent listening on the faces of the audience followed usually by laughter when the appropriate links are made.

Leeds (1988) lists no fewer than 14 devices for making an initial impact. Strategies such as audience compliment, startling statement or statistic, joke and personal experience can be useful. Equally, it is important to avoid openings that offer an apology, an explanation of your presence or how difficult you have found it to choose your topic, which detracts from the vital nature of what you are about to say. Leeds suggests that you hook your listeners at the outset; then you are well on your way to winning the battle for their attention and at the very least, you will have aroused enough curiosity that they will want to see what comes next.

KEEPING THE MATERIAL INTERESTING

This is perhaps a logical extension of the previous issue. This all depends upon the number of people involved but one way of making things interesting is to involve the audience with what is happening. People are naturally more interested in material to which they can relate and even contribute and their involvement has the added bonus of valuing their opinions and ideas.

If you feel this is not possible owing to the size of the group (although it has been claimed that buzz groups can include up to 200 delegates), try to incorporate items of everyday life such as television programmes, particularly the soaps which reflect societal issues, recent news events of an impact which most of the audience are likely to be aware of, personal experiences which demonstrate fallibility, amusing or insightful revelations which have occurred to you or people you know.

People generally relate to simple things such as common experience, a story, a familiar saying or the stimulating words of a mutually admired person. As a speaker, you are the catalyst that brings together an audience and a subject.

Cole (1993) suggested the following code of good practice in the making of presentations.

- Consider your audience and their needs.
- Assemble your facts and ideas in the light of this need and take into account the complexity of the material.

123

Six Steps to **Effective Management**

- Develop sufficient and suitable visual aids.
- Consider what other information should be made available (drawings, reports, etc.).
- Tell your audience what you are going to tell them, tell them and then tell them what you have told them!
- Be enthusiastic about the subject (unless this would be completely inappropriate, e.g. the announcement of a new redundancy plan).
- Be natural.
- Maintain eye contact with your audience.
- Be prepared for questions both during and at the end of your presentation.

MANAGEMENT OF SELF

That an audience has an effect upon how we perform is something which is explored in psychology under the term 'social facilitation' and this theory would suggest that our performance is enhanced by having an audience, especially when we are performing well known or practised functions.

However, the area which appears to cause problems for most people is that of overcoming nerves or anxiety associated with speaking in public. This is quite a natural reaction in that for most of our life we have striven to be physically and psychologically safe and in offering our ideas and thoughts in a public arena, we give others the opportunity to comment on them and perhaps ridicule or disregard them. It occurs less frequently to us that our ideas will be praised or regarded highly.

If you have sound knowledge, have prepared well and have practised or rehearsed your presentation then your confidence will be boosted. Sometimes, however, you have developed habits or defence strategies which prevent you from speaking out in an assertive or authoritative manner.

Carnegie (1990) tells the story of a board chairman who approached him because he had been terrified for years of speaking in front of others, even those he knew. He felt his problem was so severe that he was beyond help. He had come along simply because he had witnessed the transformation in one of his employees who for years had sneaked about the place with head down and eyes averted. Suddenly he walked with his chin up, a light in his eye and said 'good morning' with confidence and spirit. He had attended a course on public speaking and had obviously taken on board what he had learned.

You can use some of the strategies in Application 6.1 to reduce and manage your own tension. It is important to differentiate between nerves and tension. Nerves are essential to set the adrenaline flowing and those in the public domain will tell you that the time to worry is when you do not get nervous. Tension, however, can wreck your performance. It constricts your voice, prevents breath control and makes you look anywhere but at the audience. Clinging to a lectern or a piece of furniture, swaying, fidgeting and other distracting mannerisms are further manifestations.

Try the exercises given to control and eliminate tension and a few minutes' practice a day will eventually enable you to relax at will and, by exercising self-control, you will give an appearance of relaxed authority.

Bower (1986) offers some useful tips on using positive thoughts as opposed to self-defeating negative thoughts to help you succeed and suggests these are used while preparing the speech, approaching the day of the speech, practising the speech, while speaking to an audience and after speaking.

INTERACTIONS WITH THE MEDIA

Within the context of this chapter, the term 'media' will be treated very broadly. Using the prefix 'the' and sometimes 'mass' the term usually refers to newspapers, television and radio and other national publications. If anxiety is experienced when talking to a group of people, this can be much worse when faced with the media.

The press is important to any company or organisation, because in so many cases it serves as the communication link between you and your customers. Often what reporters write about is negative because bad things make news and this is where unfriendly feelings can build up in your relationship with the media and spoil your ability to communicate. Reporters are likely to produce a story anyway, so it is important that you ensure that it is the one you want published and this, as with all other presentation opportunities, is better for planning if at all possible.

Petersen & Hillkirk (1991) suggest that if you keep your employees well abreast of issues that the organisation faces, you can then trust them to express themselves well in whatever way comes naturally to them. An open approach to the media is always the best policy, wherever possible empowering people lower down in the organisation to act as spokespersons.

In practice, most large organisations have press and/or public relations officers who are employed to make statements to the press. Many involved in the health services are concerned about how the

Presentations to groups

future will shape up as a result of increasing evidence that the NHS is being required to preach the government 'message' (Lyall 1997). This aside, it is perhaps unlikely and definitely unwise for the un-initiated to respond to the mass media.

A salutary lesson may be learned from something which occurred in the run-up to the last election when a mundane and routine story of everyday life in the NHS was transformed by political spin-doctoring into a major election issue. A chief executive speaking at the IHSM Conference advised 'Never say "no comment", never lie and give it straight with the facts'. He continued: 'If a crisis breaks, don't say you're in a meeting, hold a press conference; being open and upfront is a better way of dealing with it' (Cervi 1997).

Media in the context of this chapter covers conference papers and display events, writing for professional journals, writing for publication in books and speaking at local fundraising events or local charitable organisations.

When preparing written or oral material for specific events or publications, it is vital to observe the instructions of the host organisation. If this is not done then however wonderful the material is, it will not be accepted or perhaps not even read. The *Health Service Journal*, for example, has some very specific guidelines regarding articles submitted and will not consider any which do not conform to these. Most conference organisers, editors, publishers and the like have more material than they can use and the first weeding out procedure might very well be whether or not the criteria for submission have been followed.

To sum up: be prepared, be honest, plan as far in advance as possible and meet the criteria of the host organisation. In this way you are less likely to experience difficulties with the media.

CONCLUSION

This chapter has shown that there are many aspects to giving presentations to groups and that, as with other skills, the more you practise, the more adept you are likely to become.

Sanders (1992) summarises his chapter on effective speaking with this list of key points which would be a useful strategy to follow.

1. Make the best of yourself.

   - Control nerves and eliminate tension
   - Share your personality
   - Stand and sit to advantage
   - Make eye contact with your audience

Communication in organisations

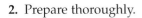

2. Prepare thoroughly.

- Realise your aim
- Know your audience
- Select and organise your material
- Shape your talk

3. Explore the full potential of your voice.

- Practise breath control
- Achieve full resonance
- Articulate (the way you say things)
- Modulate (the pace at which you say things)

Giving presentations or speaking in public can be an invigorating and worthwhile exercise which enhances your professional and personal skill base.

Practice checklist

The following checklist indicates how you can use in your practice the issues discussed in this chapter by asking yourself the following questions.

- Have I prepared my material well?
- Do I know my subject?
- Have I found out as much as I can about the venue?
- Am I using my visual material as an aid or a crutch?
- Does the material I am presenting make sense?
- Am I able to be flexible whilst following my plan?
- Have I considered the audience?
- Am I able to accept that it may not go perfectly?
- Am I willing to make allowances for myself?
- Can I deal with any feedback I get?

Discussion questions

- What are the most frequent barriers to effective interaction in a presentation scenario?
- Discuss the visual aids you would use for a humorous and informative presentation on the pitfalls of visual aids. Try to sketch them out and show how you would make each point.

Presentations to groups

Communication in organisations

(Cont.)

- You have been chosen to introduce your Head of Department (HOD) at an employee orientation programme. Discuss what would contribute to a powerful introduction which will make both you and your HOD look good.
- Your topic is Health for All in the 21st Century. Devise four different openings using the following attention-getters: a joke, a rhetorical question, a startling statistic and a personal story.

References

Bower S 1986 Painless public speaking. Thorsons, New York

Carnegie D 1990 Quick and easy ways to effective speaking. Pocketbooks, New York

Cervi B 1997 The perils of playing it by ear. Health Service Journal 107: 10

Cole GA 1993 Management theory and practice, 4th edn. DP Publications, London

Leeds D 1988 Powerspeak – the complete guide to public speaking and presentation. Piatkus, London

Lyall J 1997 Future tense. News Focus. Health Service Journal 107: 5

Petersen D, Hillkirk J 1991 Teamwork – new management ideas for the 90s. Gollancz, London

Sanders B 1992 Effective speaking. In: Stewart DM (ed) Handbook of management skills. Gower, London

Stewart DM (ed) 1992 Handbook of management skills. Gower, London

Walklin L 1990 Teaching and learning in further and adult education. Stanley Thornes, Cheltenham

Further reading

Bellamy K 1995 Design standards for computer generated teaching slides. Journal of Audiovisual Media in Medicine 18(3): 115–120
Reports on a study undertaken on the slide-making habits of professional health care educators and common problems in design capability are identified and addressed.

Bower S 1986 Painless public speaking. Thorsons, New York
A mixture of practical advice and psychological support using illustrative triggers to structure the text. Includes a number of speaking techniques to increase impact.

Johns M 1995 Design for slides. Journal of Audiovisual Media in Medicine 18(3): 121–128
Looks at the basic principles of design for projection slides and in particular those produced on a personal computer and destined to be used for a meeting or seminar.

Kirsta A 1986 The book of stress survival. Guild, London
Covers a wide range of strategies to combat stress and live positively but included here primarily for its relatively extensive range of simple relaxation exercises.

Moore W 1997 My word. Health Service Journal 107: 26–27
This article publicises writers in the NHS and gives some tips on what publishers want, with details of a King's Fund step-by-step guide to producing a book proposal.

Rae L 1983 The skills of training: a guide for managers and practitioners. Gower Business Studies, Aldershot
Although this book is written from a training perspective, Chapter 2 contains some useful information on the advantages and disadvantages of the lecture.

Turner S 1994 The public speaker's companion. Thorsons, London
A relatively light-hearted look at speaking on all, including social, occasions but nevertheless contains a large number of tried and tested hints and tips for the would-be public speaker.

Presentations to groups

Application **6:1**

Brenda Maslen

Developing your presentation skills

Communication in organisations

It will be essential for you to apply the information contained in this chapter to your own working life, selecting areas which are most pertinent to yourself and discarding those which you do not find helpful. Many people who make their living from public speaking, some of whom are in the list of further reading, suggest that if you follow some simple rules, you too will be able to master the art. The following activities suggest ways in which you could structure this activity.

One way in which you can develop your expertise in this area, or indeed any other, is to develop a personal action plan. It can take any format you wish but it needs to identify your aims, where you currently are and where you would like to be. You should set yourself a time limit in order to maintain motivation. It could look something like this.

Outcome

1. Identify venues available to me for presentation purposes.
2. Develop material to support my presentation.
3. Manage my own anxiety when thinking of speaking in front of an audience.
4. Add any other outcomes you wish.

Now ask yourself whether you have achieved this outcome fully, almost, partly or not at all and identify the action you will now take.

- I need to develop my knowledge base in:
- I need to develop my skill base in:
- This is who I think can help me:
- These are the other resources I need to achieve my outcomes:
- I will make another plan by: (date)
- I will achieve my outcomes by: (date)

Look at this example from Castling (1996). Although she is writing specifically about teaching and training, the information

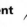

has a wider application. Think back to occasions when you were being talked or lectured at and try to recall aspects which prevented you gaining as much as you could from the event. Compile a list of what went wrong and then compare it with the following.

- Room stuffy, poor ventilation, too small for size of audience
- Hard chairs
- Speaker went far too fast
- A lot of this went over my head
- Speaker didn't check what we already knew
- Monotonous voice, I lost interest
- Used jargon without explanation
- Why are senior managers always described as 'he'?
- Hardly ever looked at my side of the room
- Used lots of clichés and kept saying 'OK'
- Couldn't see visual aids, writing too small, colours faint
- Gave us a 10-page handout, I needn't have come
- Seemed to be all over the place, no structure

A similar type of checklist is included in Rae (1983) when writing of the lecture as a form of training.

1. The lecturer has:
- low skills in the art of public speaking
- prepared the material badly and it may not all be relevant
- presented the material in an unorganised way.

2. The lecture:
- contains too much, too complex material to readily assimilate.

3. The audience:
- is asked to do no more than appear to be listening and thus is allowed to be completely passive.

You could perhaps measure your own performance against these categories or get a friend to do so and then see where your strengths lie and what areas would benefit from some development and then use a personal action plan to work on these.

A preparation checklist might help you to ensure that you have structured the work in the most effective way. These are the areas you might like to address.

Structure

- Does your OPENING contain an outline of the material, set the context and state your outcomes?
- What are the main points you want to make?
- Do they follow each other logically, linking together well?
- Are they well 'signposted', covering the material you want to cover?

Developing your presentation skills

131

- Do they need support from visual aids?
- When CLOSING do you sum up the main points and make a strong conclusion?

Delivery

- Do you know your presentation? Are you going to use cue cards?
- What will be your position – are you going to sit or stand?
- Who will you make eye contact with?
- Is the language you are going to use right for your audience?
- Do you know how to use your visual aids?

Visual aids

- Are your aids simple, interesting and easy to read?
- Do they fit well with your talk and add to your presentation?

Question handling

- Are you knowledgeable in your subject?
- Can you anticipate and prepare for any likely questions?
- Do you think you can answer any questions clearly?

To discover the importance of being specific and the uniqueness of each individual, reflect upon the example given from Walklin at the beginning of the section on audiovisual aids (p. 120) and then extend it by describing something to which a name can be put, say for example a house or a car, and then ask one member of the group to describe the house or car they have imagined and await the chorus of alternatives which is likely to follow. This shows how shared concepts are interpreted differently by each individual. It follows that being specific is very important so if you want your audience to imagine something, tell them exactly what it is, for

(p. 120)

Box 6.1.1

Non-projected aids	*Projected aids*	*Audio aids*
Chalkboard	Overhead projector	Cassette tapes
Markerboard	35 mm slides	Compact discs
The real thing	Closed circuit TV	Audio tapes
Models	Video	
Charts	Television	
Posters	Computer-generated material	

Box 6.1.2	Evaluation	
Aid	*Why effective*	*Limitation*

example a small thatched cottage with roses round the door or a long, black, sleek Jaguar car.

On the topic of using audio, projected visual aids and non-projected visual aids, look at the most commonly used aids listed in Box 6.1 and then work with the evaluation sheet (Box 6.2) to analyse their strengths and limitations.

In order to demonstrate how emphasis and attitude can affect your voice, try the following activity. Say 'well' as if you were:

- annoyed
- disgusted
- surprised
- thrilled
- in doubt
- suspicious
- thoughtful
- pugnacious.

If you find this useful there are many other vocal exercises in Dorothy Leeds' book from which this is reproduced.

In order to be successful in giving talks or offering expert opinion, you could try a little supportive self-talk and mental rehearsal. Ask yourself the following questions.

- Where did you first get the idea that your thoughts and feelings were any less important than anyone else's?
- Is there any objective reason to continue to believe this now?
- What communication habits have you fallen into to protect yourself in situations that intimidate you?

Now close your eyes and imagine a situation in which you are required to present some information and look at the thoughts and feelings that accompany this. Move through the scenario to where you see yourself walking briskly on to the platform, smiling and addressing the audience in a confident and relaxed manner, dealing with questions from the floor including those to which you have no specific answer, concluding your talk and leaving the platform to tumultuous applause.

What were your feelings when you imagined yourself acting confidently in this situation? You may conclude after doing this exercise and perhaps repeating it a number of times that reality is likely to mirror your imagination.

To continue this theme there are a number of exercises which, when used on a daily basis, will enable you to relax at will. The following simple breathing exercise may stimulate you to use others.

When you are feeling tense try this tranquillising exercise.

1. Breathe in through the nose to a slow, steady count of four. As your lung capacity improves, increase the count to six or eight. Hold your breath for a further count of four, six or eight.
2. Without moving your body, begin to breathe out to a slow, steady count of four, six or eight. Expel all the air completely. After the last number, begin again.

Feedback has only been mentioned briefly but it is vital in every form of interaction in order for you to develop your expertise. When asking for feedback, be careful not to include categories which are beyond your control or which cannot be altered. Evaluation has been given some bad press by this type of activity, making it appear to be merely a paper exercise.

You might like to develop your own feedback forms along the lines of the major categories mentioned in the preparation checklist. The responses requested may be fairly generalised, which is likely to result in qualitative data, or you may wish to be more specific and design a numerical scale which is likely to result in quantitative data. Perhaps a mixture of the two is best.

A blend of knowledge, skills and attitudes enables you to approach this important area of expertise with confidence and enthusiasm for your topic will reduce the anxiety you feel in addressing others. Perhaps Bower (1986) summed it up most pertinently with the following:

Courage comes from **wanting** to say it well.

Security comes from **knowing** you can say it well.

Confidence comes from **having** said it well.

References

Bower S 1986 Painless public speaking. Thorsons, New York

Castling A 1996 Competence-based teaching and training. Macmillan, Basingstoke

Rae L 1983 The skills of training: a guide for managers and practitioners. Gower Business Studies, Aldershot

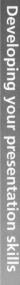

Developing your presentation skills

Chapter **Seven**

Networking

Colleen Wedderburn Tate

- ● **Groups and group theory**
- ● **Your membership of groups and their value to you**
- ● **Types of networks**
- ● **How to network**
- ● **Active networking**
- ● **Related issues**

O V E R V I E W

Most of us are born into networks called families. Whether through technology or alliances, we are all becoming part of larger networks. To remain unaware of this is to risk being left out of key activities which affect work and personal life. This chapter describes the significance and relevance of human networks and suggests ways to become successful and remain so within them.

With the significance of professional networks becoming more pervasive in the NHS, particularly in relation to senior appointments, it is becoming very important to access and use the opportunities afforded through wide contact with many people. Even if you do not wish to gain rapid promotion, the need to be effective in the professional and managerial network in your place of work is crucial if you are to be effective in your role. Putting aside such political and professional aspirations, it is also clear that the world of health care is so complex now that it is impossible to rely on a small circle of colleagues for support and advice. This chapter is therefore an important aspect of communication in a complex world.

Some theory is provided in the Application as a conceptual framework while practical and anecdotal elements are included to relate this to the reality of everyday life as a clinical professional and manager. It is intended that, with the main chapter, these should give you the basic knowledge required to start building a network and to be confident in doing this.

INTRODUCTION

Networking is a communication process, the aim being to meet and get to know people from diverse backgrounds. One expectation is that you may be helpful to them and they may be helpful to you at some point in the future. Like any form of communication, to be successful, networking needs to be selective to ensure accuracy, relevance and interest. If you were to network with every person you met, your networks might be huge but of little benefit to you or others in the network. There are different styles of networking, one of which, the open style, appears to be random and is difficult to keep focused. (Networking styles are discussed below.) But even the most inveterate open networker can only keep in touch with a limited number of people.

For most people networking begins at school, where they make choices about who they will associate with and who they will not. Playground games include a large element of group forming and group development. It is very important to children that they have friends that they like and who like them. As we grow up we become more sophisticated about choosing who we associate with. Most teenagers leave school or college with a set of friends and acquaintances who may continue to be part of their network for some time. This group formation and development process is encouraged by many schools with alumni associations, ex-pupils being encouraged to return and help the school and students, even more so if the old girl or boy has reached a position of power and influence. In some educational establishments there is a great deal of emphasis on networking and the benefits of being 'in the club' seem to be great. But it can also create anxiety, tension and a feeling of being excluded; many of us have experience of feeling not part of the 'in' crowd. Such feelings can be exacerbated if, as part of your job, you have to meet and communicate with many people. Therefore it is important to realise that networking is a skill that requires practice and development and, if necessary, rehearsal.

It is in the workplace that networking becomes a blessing and a curse. For nurses, many of whom still enter their initial education course straight from school, two networks are of immediate importance: people in college and those met during clinical placements.

Someone once said that the friends you make in nursing or other health care professions are for life. This may not be far from the truth. Networks consist of people who share common interests. People tend to mix with people they are most comfortable with and, often, social friends are also work colleagues. How many of your social contacts did you first meet in the work environment? Furthermore, nursing and other clinical professions are part of a huge international profession. Under such circumstances, it is almost impossible not to network. It is more probable that we do not take advantage of the opportunities to network.

GROUPS AND GROUP THEORY

Those people who become long-term network members are often the ones who have gone through a process of learning together. Tuckman (1965) looks at group development in detail. Aspects of a typical group development process based on Tuckman's work might be as shown in Table 7.1.

There is no requirement to go through each stage. For example, the storming stage might not take place or a group might never get to the performing stage. For the purposes of understanding the relevance to networking, the columns headed *Relationship behaviour* and *Relationship outcome* are the most important. If people participate in a process that moves from dependency to hostility, cohesion and interdependence, then it is likely that disengagement will only be partial. If relationship outcomes have moved through acceptance, belonging, support, pride and satisfaction, then it is likely that individuals are going to want to repeat that relationship. This is a promising start of a network of like-minded people who know each other's strengths and weaknesses. Another way of looking at this model would be to say that the task is building relationships between group members and the 'performing' aspect is a successful lasting network. The adjourning stage might not be for 50 years or more!

There are many people with whom you might network but may never work with. For example, someone at a conference with whom you have a brief conversation and swap business cards could be as important a member of your network as someone you have worked closely with over a period of years. The group processes at conferences may seem artificial, but nevertheless can be very powerful in terms of your future development.

Table 7.1 Aspects of the group development process (adapted from Tuckman 1965)

Process stage	Task behaviour	Relationship behaviour	General theme	Task outcome	Relationship outcome
Forming	Orientation	Dependency	Awareness	Commitment	Acceptance
Storming	Resistance	Hostility	Conflict	Clarification	Belonging
Norming	Communication	Cohesion	Cooperation	Involvement	Support
Performing	Problem solving	Interdependence	Productivity	Achievement	Pride
Adjourning	Termination	Disengagement	Separation	Recognition	Satisfaction

Networking

Where work and professional meetings differ is in the reciprocity needed to maintain work relationships. Both environments may provide networking opportunities but work also demands that networks benefit you and the organisation you work with – for example, working in partnership with another department or even another organisation. Deffenbaugh (2001) argues that the NHS has a self-contained 'silo' mentality that prevents an integrated approach to planning and delivering services. It is fair to say the NHS has, in the past, been very introverted and reluctant to 'think outside the box'. Even organisations need to network, if only to prevent themselves from reinventing wheels. Neither organisations nor individuals can any longer afford to 'go it alone'. Networks contain information, support, knowledge and, ultimately, power.

YOUR MEMBERSHIP OF GROUPS AND THEIR VALUE TO YOU

Some people who have very technical jobs think that knowledge of the tasks is enough and people should respect knowledgeable individuals and cooperate with them in the workplace. But it is not enough to be technically competent if other people are reluctant to work with you. Many of the solutions to complex problems rely on informal contacts to get information or assistance that is not readily available from within formal resources. Those who develop a network of people who provide this informal extra resource become more successful than others and are seen as people to associate with. Most people realise that there is some truth in the saying 'It's not what you know that matters but who you know'. As the individual becomes more skilled at networking so they become more confident and more competent (that is, they know more, are better informed and communicate more effectively).

One example of this virtuous circle is the job interview. The vacancy may have been advertised, been heard of through word of mouth or seen on the Internet. You might be one of several candidates who meet the personnel specification and are competent to do the job. But what if one of the other candidates used their network to find out information about the organisation that was not in the information pack sent to applicants? That person would certainly have a head start. This scenario is becoming more common, especially for senior positions. It is no longer enough to complete the application form and wait for a response. Consider your own reactions to two people, one whom you have just met for the first time and someone you met a year ago and had a 5-minute conversation with. Although you do not know the latter person well, you have probably already formed a strong opinion of them. Do you like them? Are they knowledgeable? Would you want to work with them? Are they your 'kind of person'?

Typically, we form opinions about people within one minute of meeting them. That opinion tends to be reinforced over time, sometimes disregarding information that might conflict with it. Unless we are perverse, we can use our network to check or challenge our opinion or get support for it. Conversely, you can use your network to ensure that you get the referees who will be most beneficial to your application. Some references are more equal than others.

So is this type of networking honest and fair? If you have derived benefit from networks you will probably believe that it is acceptable. If you had negative experiences you will probably stop reading about here. It really does not matter what you answered. The end result is the only way of measuring the validity of networking. Most organisations do not employ people who cannot do their job. It is in their interest to have bright, enthusiastic people, so be clear – networking can only get you through the door. What you do when you get there will be a combination of your skills, your understanding of the function of networks and self-belief.

Of course, there are limits to how far people can network. You can try and network with knowledgeable, influential people with whom you have little in common but networking is a two-way process. It requires practice and knowing how to network and what types of networks are available.

TYPES OF NETWORKS

Michelli & Straw (1995) considered the types of networks to be:

- personal
- professional
- organisational
- strategic.

The first two are primarily focused on you, the last two are primarily about developing organisations. However, you may have international networks which are more important to you than local or professional ones.

Personal networks

Simply put, these are school friends, family, colleagues and even your boss who may all be part of your personal network. You never

Networking

lose your personal networks and they remain important throughout your life. Personal networks consist of people who you choose to spend your time with. Like all networks, they need investment, commitment, attention and development. Personal networks can provide you with employment, support, acceptance and information.

Professional networks

These networks can be powerful aids to your development. They provide information, influence, development and support. They are also global and can provide links to other networks; for example, the Royal Colleges of Nursing and Midwifery are linked to the World Health Organization. Some professional groups are part of the national and by definition the international trade union movement. Professional networks can be intraorganisational (the grapevine, personal alliances) or extraorganisational (alumni associations, past colleagues, competitors). After personal networks, they are your most important network, as well as your largest.

Organisational networks

This is the informal part of the organisation. Who talks to whom? Who eats with whom? You may already be aware that the real power in your organisation does not necessarily lie with senior managers. 'Hubs' – people who know what's really going on, who have influence (personal power) and who get things done – are the true sources of power. They may not hold senior positions or long tenure, but they are natural networkers. When you go to a new job or organisation, take the time to identify the 'hubs'. It will also give you practice in observing how organisations really work, at the informal level.

Strategic networks

These are groups of organisations with a common purpose. You might believe that this describes the NHS but NHS trusts specifically are, in the main, vertically integrated organisations – hierarchical and inward looking with set methods and procedures. A strategic alliance of organisations creates more flexibility and, in an ideal world, shares risk. The PFI initiatives, planned partnerships with the private sector, services such as NHS Direct and some

Communication in organisations

aspects of telemedicine are examples of how health services in the UK are becoming disintegrated and, in the future, probably virtual. You therefore need to develop skills to work in these new organisations – effective networking being one.

HOW TO NETWORK

First, you need to map your network. Who's in it? What kind of network is it? To help you, draw a circle. Put your name in the circle and draw another circle attached to the first one by a straight line. In this second circle put the name of one of your networks (personal, etc.). Attach as many circles to this second circle as you like to represent the people in the network (again, link with straight lines). If you met an individual through another person in the network, join these by a hatch line. When you've finished you'll have a diagram that looks like a mind map or a tree. As you develop your networking skills, this map will change. Networks need nurturing and feeding or they will die.

Second, you need to determine your networking style. There are three styles.

Conscious networkers

These people have clear goals, know they have gaps in their networks and find ways and people to fill them. You would adopt this style if you were particularly concerned with developing and advancing your career.

Open networkers

These people value networks for their future potential. They sometimes find it difficult to be focused because they have no immediate goal in mind. You may have this style if you tend to network for its own sake.

Intuitive networkers

Altruism is a driver for these networkers. They are drawn by common values and have strong networks. Intuitive networkers sometimes do not benefit personally from their activities, although others do.

Networking

143

ACTIVE NETWORKING

At work

In the work environment it is worth considering the different groupings of individuals. There is a tendency for people to develop closer working relationships with others in the same ward, department or profession. You might want to increase the range of your network members by including others outside those circles. Where are the opportunities to do so? Volunteering for work on committees is one way of increasing the range of people you come into contact with. This has a potentially negative effect in that, by attending meetings, you have less time to get the job done. However, successful networking will enable you to do your job better using the informal network to gain information and speed up the decision making processes. The time spent networking will save time in other parts of the job and the net effect will be positive. The process of networking itself makes a job more interesting and that is likely to have performance benefits.

In your professions

Within nursing and other clinical professions there is ample scope to network. Many people start by going to conferences and although it may be daunting to go up to a complete stranger and say 'Hello, I don't know anyone here, can I introduce myself?', it becomes easier once you have done it the first time. It is surprising how many people are too shy to strike up a conversation with strangers but are pleased to meet someone new in that sort of environment. It is also useful to remember to thank conference speakers, take their card and follow up conversations if necessary. They are more likely to remember you at a future meeting. However, you should resist becoming a 'professional conference attendee'. Like networks, choose your conferences with care.

In your trade union/professional organisation

Joining a professional organisation can be a good way to increase your network very quickly. If you operate at local level then you will be involved in joint staff consultative committees and assisting others with work-related problems. You will mix with groups of people who you do not normally meet in a working week. This is

Communication in organisations

a valuable opportunity to meet and work with senior managers in a way that allows for greater understanding of each other's strengths and helps to build mutual respect. However, some work colleagues will feel you are deserting them by fraternising with the management and you will need to be careful to explain the benefits of working in this way. There is no point in gaining valuable contacts in one area only to lose them in another.

Annual conferences are an ideal place to meet people. You do not need to be a delegate from your local branch, although that helps. To increase your profile, try to talk to the conference from the podium and you will find people stopping you for a chat afterwards. There are often fringe meetings at conferences that are worth attending as, again, this broadens the group of people that you meet face to face. When you go for the second year you will be able to renew acquaintances quickly and easily.

Subprofessional interest groups

Some professional organisations have specialist interest groups. Often there is a section for managers which is a very useful networking environment. If you are spending time with a group with narrow interests – perhaps a clinical specialist group – then be aware that you also need to be involved with other groups to balance this.

Newsletters

Increasingly, organisations are using newsletters as a formal network and they encourage staff to become more involved at work. The best newsletters provide information speedily, allow members to display their own messages and invite people to participate in activities where there are greater opportunities to network individually. If your organisation has a newsletter, do you write for it? Offer to edit it? Take a 'vox pop' slot? This will enable you to express rationally based personal opinion on work or professional issues which might get you noticed. Any of these activities will increase your visibility in the organisation (if that's what you want), improve your communication skills and increase your information.

Internet

The Internet has a multitude of bulletin boards which are changing and being added to all the time. But beware – if you give out your email address on one of these you will probably be flooded with replies, some of which will be inappropriate. If you shy away from the Internet because it involves using a computer, think of it as just another way to write a letter. As far as your career is concerned, you can apply on-line for a host of jobs and even be interviewed on-line. This is impersonal but better than the artificial nature of a face-to-face interview and has the remarkable benefit of displaying your cyber skills to a potential employer (see Chapter Ten for more on this form of networking).

Dinner parties

People who host dinner parties are social 'introducers' who hopefully can cook or have access to someone who can! It is usually people who are good at networking already who run this sort of social event so if you want to develop your networking skills, attend one, observe and ask questions. The technique is to invite people from diverse backgrounds so that conversations can be wide ranging. If the people invited all work together it should come as no surprise if they talk shop all evening. Inviting people to dinner often results in you being invited to other parties where you have opportunities to develop your own network.

Courses

Like conferences, be discriminating. What is the value of a course to you? Do you spend time and money to increase your knowledge of a particular topic only? Many people see the benefit of a course as not only the knowledge gained but also the interesting people you meet on the course. These two aspects are evenly balanced. You might want to find out who else is going on a course before you commit yourself. It may be better use of your time to attend courses where you can gain both knowledge and networking contacts at the same time. Ask for the statistics of the course – pass rate, testimonials from past attendees, audit results, background and expertise of the tutors. Well-run courses will have all this information and more. If some of it is not available, think twice.

Scholarships, travel awards and bursaries, international fellowships and secondments are also valuable. There are numerous awards for health care workers, many of which are available to nurses, midwives and health visitors. The author's personal experience of receiving such awards has proved the benefits – living in a different country, learning to communicate in another language, sharing skills and ideas, and developing new networks. The benefits far outweigh the disadvantages (being away from familiar surroundings being the biggest). Such time-outs and secondments are finally becoming accepted in the NHS and are a key part of career development of future senior managers and chief executives.

Journal groups

A journal group is a meeting, usually informal, of individuals who have an interest in a common topic. It could be a group of managers interested in developing their management knowledge. Each person in the group agrees to read a particular journal on a regular basis and then present a summary of the relevant information from that journal to the group. This idea has two purposes. First, it enables individuals to gain a wider knowledge of written material than they would have time to read themselves. Second, the discussion following the presentations allows networking to take place. Once a group is formed and seen as useful, it is surprising how quickly others want to join in. It helps the forming process if the group meets at lunchtime and food is provided although this is not essential.

Writing for publication

Someone once said that we all have at least one book in us. When it comes to articles we have several. Every professional journal includes a 'writing for publication' page. There are several writing workshops specifically designed for nurses, midwives and health visitors and many innovations and initiatives to share through journal pages. If you do not feel up to writing an article, use the letters pages or submit a short piece on your personal view of a small aspect of health care (always write from the heart with your head firmly screwed on). You'll get to see your name in print and, best of all, you may find others who agree with you. But a caveat – once you start, you won't want to stop.

RELATED ISSUES

Gender

Gender does have an impact on networking. Do you network better with men or women? What are the reasons for this and should

Networking

you make a special effort to change this pattern? Do men and women network in different ways? There are no simple answers to these questions but personal experience suggests that women seem to be intuitive networkers while men appear to be conscious networkers. Given that conscious networking is more targeted and deliberate, it may not appeal to women. But the altruism implied in intuitive networking may not be the most effective policy for women who seek career advancement.

Race and religion

In a recent article in the *Harvard Business Review*, David A Thomas (2001) argues that race is a factor in mentoring ethnic minorities. Members of ethnic minority groups, at least in corporate America, are late developers, career advancement coming after they have reached middle management. Significantly, their success correlates with having a 'strong network of mentors and corporate sponsors' (Thomas 2001). Their white counterparts tend to progress much more quickly from the start. Might there be differences in how white and black nurses network and differences in their experiences? Might differences exist in terms of religion? Certainly networking is seen as an important skill in Western society but it is also important in other societies, with the family playing a central role. Many religious groups network among their own members, sometimes to the exclusion of those outside. These can be useful groups, especially if they are diverse in terms of individuals' backgrounds, upbringing, employment and interests.

Social class

Every society has some kind of class system. Networking according to class exists in North America, the UK and parts of the Caribbean. This falls into the category of personal networks, but can be a source of power and influence. Such networks tend to be exclusive and selective. Membership is based on a variety of factors – the type of school or university a person attended, money, influence, family connection or notoriety.

CONCLUSION

Networking is a lifelong activity. Your aim is to make and maintain a set of contacts that guarantees you have someone to consult on any topic at any time. Those contacts will themselves have networks of people who may be available to you and so become part of your network. The earlier you start, the wider and the more successful the network will be. But it's never too late to start. If you have not already built up a sizeable network, map one out and begin the process. Perhaps in a few years' time you will be the person who enters a room and knows most of the people there. You will be able to renew acquaintances, reinforce the strength of your network and enable others to do the same.

Practice checklist

- If you haven't already done so, join a network, referring to the network types on pp. 141–143. Which networks are right for you now?
- When you read journals, note those organisations (not necessarily hospitals) which are doing interesting things. Call and speak to the person or people mentioned in the article or news story. This serves at least three purposes: they will be pleased at your interest, you will have increased your network by at least one person and it will build your confidence for future networking. You can use a similar method with speakers at conferences who often are not fully acknowledged for their talk. In either case, be sincere and honest.
- If you have never been to a reunion of your school or college, go to the next one. Better still, organise one yourself. Who knows, your next job may come from it.
- If you're an active networker already, review what you're doing and how you're doing it. Networks are like gardens – pruning and variety make for better displays.

Discussion questions

- To network effectively requires a certain amount of assertive behaviour. Look again at the barriers to assertiveness on p. 18. Do any of these barriers apply to how you approach networking?
- The concept of the 'old boy network' has probably caused many people to shy away from networks. Is this your experience? If it has been, can you now see how networks can be positive? If you network actively, how do you alter some of your colleagues' beliefs that networks are for the elite?

Networking

References

Deffenbaugh J 2001 Coming up for air. Health Service Journal 111(5753): 31

Michelli D, Straw A 1995 Successful networking in a week.
Headway/Hodder and Stoughton, London

Thomas DA 2001 The truth about mentoring minorities: race matters.
Harvard Business Review April: 98–107

Tuckman B 1965 Developmental sequences in small groups. Psychological
Bulletin 63(6): 384–399

Further reading

Michelli D, Straw A 1995 Successful networking in a week. Headway/
Hodder and Stoughton, London

Communication in organisations

Application **7:1**

Colleen Wedderburn Tate

A personal exercise

The following is an exercise you might conduct using some of the thoughts presented in this chapter. What groups are you a part of and how do you network with the people in them?

As you meet more and more people you may develop a strategy for deciding if someone is going to be useful in your network. Consider writing down how people connect with you and link this to yourself in terms of professional, personal and career development. Does any of this assist your goals in these areas?

There will be too many meetings to include everybody. Who should you include and who should you, reluctantly, exclude? It is tempting to say that people in the same line of work or with the same interests are the most important. I suggest that you consider your network as a means of broadening your knowledge. You should include anyone who is interesting no matter what their knowledge and interests are. As your career progresses there is no guarantee that you will remain in the same field of work. Many people have career changes and as society develops it seems that this is becoming more likely. Even if you do not change careers it is amazing how much people from other disciplines can contribute to your problem solving and decision making.

Application 7:2
Mark Darley

How networking might assist career development: a fictional example

Mary Nightingale qualified in a health care profession in 1975. At the time personal networks were strong but professional ones were nascent. Mary joined the professional body/trade union for her clinical profession. As a student she was locally active and even became involved in national matters, taking the consequent opportunity to attend conferences.

Although Mary was at an early part of her career she was noticed and given an invitation to undertake specialist training. This was accepted and she began a course in a specialist area of care at a leading London hospital. During this time a number of important projects were successfully concluded, some of which were written up in professional journals.

After 3 years of clinical work Mary took the chance to become part of the clinical management team after someone was promoted. At the time she was completing a Masters degree in a non-clinical subject which had managerial relevance. This was followed by 4 years working at a senior level gaining valuable experience, after which ambition dictated that it was time to look for a position closer to board level. While this was not an explicit wish from the outset, the desire to contribute in this way grew with changes in the NHS which presented non-medical clinicians with chances to progress managerially.

After two attempts Mary was successful in gaining a position in a medium-sized acute hospital. This position was held for 5 years and then a directorship was advertised in the west of England for which a successful application was made. After another 4 years this hospital merged with a larger neighbour and Mary was not successful in being appointed to the new board. A move back to the south of England was made into another hospital outside the NHS.

Although the new post was not ideal, efforts to move were frustrated by the fact that the most recent experience was gained in an area geographically remote from the new one. Less experienced individuals seemed to gain preference for posts. It seemed that local profile counted for much.

- Consider the use of networks in the progress Mary made towards achieving the board appointment.
- What happened to her networks on moving south?
- What lessons might there be in this story?
- Can you think of relevant situations in your own working life where better networking might have produced better or different outcomes?

Consideration of the above points will enhance your appreciation of the importance of networks and gaining a good profile through them when seeking senior appointments in particular. Good networking skills are not a substitute for knowledge, skill and achievement but a good network can be an excellent shop window through which the profession and colleagues can gain a good impression of how you might contribute to an organisation or to a particular project.

How networking might assist career development

Application 7:3
Janet Knowles

Working in the NHS

Involvement in the NHS is about maximising the efficiency and benefit to the organisation by creating a functional network of interpersonal regard at all levels and between all colleagues. Why does this have such a good effect on the organisation?

With the pressures of the workplace today and all the conflicting attitudes and approaches, we are missing out the most powerful unifying and developmental force available to us: that of people who collude in identifying and contributing to putting in the framework to achieve a service that is as good as it can possibly be. If a network of people can be developed who are all aiming for the same goal then you have a vehicle for:

- improving individual knowledge/information
- providing relevant advice, reaction, comments and suggestions
- acting as a sounding board for clarifying ideas and strategies
- extending influence and support
- streamlining working relationships.

How, then, is it possible to practise this approach if there are people around you who seem to be working intensely to curb this team spirit for their own benefit? This certainly needs to be addressed but the most important action for you to consider is the original plan of campaign.

How then can you start to foster this approach?

COMMUNICATING INVOLVEMENT

Behind every successful strategy there is a clear plan of approach so let's identify an action plan for what you wish to achieve. First, you need to collect the information that will focus this plan. Standing where you are now:

- what are your work concerns regarding relationship issues at this time?

- go through these concerns and decide those that you can do something about and those that you cannot.

Identify your major concerns at this time. Divide them into those you can and those you cannot change or influence. Consider those you cannot influence first. Is it a personal or common frustration? Is it a major part of your life or are you making more of the problem than you need? How can you mitigate the effects of the situation so that it becomes more comfortable? In the longer term what changes can you make to your own lifestyle that will take the problem away?

Those that you cannot change or influence you have to learn to live with as comfortably as possible, so consider how this can be achieved. Just accepting that there is nothing you can radically change about the facts of an issue enables you to view this in a different light.

Those that you can influence must now be addressed.

- Identify them.

1.
2.
3.

- Take each concern in turn and analyse what you want to happen.
- Be quite hard with yourself and determine whether what you want to happen is feasible or logical.
- What would be the downside if you achieved what you wish?

1. to yourself?
2. to others?

- How would you deal with these issues?

Having evaluated the background to your target, now turn to how you intend to actually achieve it. The actual approach might include the following.

1. Who do you need to contact within the organisation to help you?
2. Is it within their power to help you in the way that you expect?
3. How do you need to put the issue to them so that they:

- understand the background to what you are asking?
- are aware of the reasons for your request?
- have a clear knowledge of the importance of the issues both to you and to the organisation?
- understand the timescales involved?

Working in the NHS

Six Steps to **Effective Management**

It is always a good idea to put some of the issues in written form; talking things through is often more negotiable but you need to have the issue in a form that can be referred to easily and that allows you to check on the existing and ongoing decisions and promises.

NEXT STEPS

Contacting people

This incorporates the need for clear and concise communication skills appropriate to the situation and the people involved.

Communication is the active involvement of at least two people in the giving and receiving of information in a variety of formats. It is certainly *not* just giving or passing out information and leaving it at that. It is the responsibility of the person giving the information to ensure that it has been received and understood in the way intended.

Every person has a particular style of communication and preference for gaining information, either verbally or visually.

What is your preferred style?

The short questionnaire below will help you to explore the strengths you use in your relationships with others. This will not only identify your own style but enable you to understand that people vary widely in how they give and receive information.

To complete this questionnaire, consider the following statements and the four different endings. Circle the statement that is most like you.

Box 7.3.1

1. I feel satisfied with myself when I:

get more things accomplished than I planned.

understand the underlying feelings of others and react in a helpful way. ⓐ

resolve a problem by using a logical, systematic method. ⓑ

develop new thoughts or ideas which can be related. ⓒ
ⓓ

2. I find it easy to be convincing when I am:

down to earth and to the point.

in touch with my own and others' feelings. ⓐ

logical and forebearing. ⓑ

intellectually on top of things and take all relevant factors into account. ⓒ
ⓓ

Ⓐ

Communication in organisations

(*Cont.*)

3. I enjoy it when others see me as:
a dependable individual who gets things done and 'comes through'. A
creative and stimulating. B
an individual who knows where he or she is going and has the
  competence to get there. C
intellectually gifted and having vision. D

**4. When confronted by others with a different point of view,
I can usually make progress by:**
getting at least one or two specific commitments on which we
  can build later. A
trying to place myself in the 'shoes of others'. B
keeping my composure and helping others to see things simply
  and logically. C
relying on my basic ability to conceptualise and pull ideas together. D

5. In time terms, I probably concentrate most on:
my immediate actions and involvements and whether they make
  sense today. A
whether what I'm doing or planning to do is going to hurt or
  disturb others. B
making sure that any actions I take are consistent and part of a
  systematic progression. C
significant long-range actions I plan to take and how they relate
  to my life's direction. D

**6. In reacting to individuals whom I meet socially,
I am likely to consider whether:**
they know what they're doing and can get things done. A
they are interesting and fun to be with. B
they seem thoughtful and reflective. C
they can contribute ideas and challenge. D

7. I am likely to impress others as being:
practical and to the point. A
sensitive and somewhat stimulating. B
astute and logical. C
intellectually oriented and somewhat complex. D

8. In the way I work on projects, I may:
want to be sure the project has a tangible 'pay-out' that will
  justify spending my time and energy on it. A
want it to be stimulating and involve lively interaction with others. B

> (*Cont.*)
>
> concentrate on making sure that the project is systematically
>   or logically developed.   C
> be most concerned as to whether the project breaks new
>   ground or advances knowledge.   D
>
> **9. In communicating with others, I may:**
> generally ignore those who talk about 'long-range implications'
>   and direct my attention to what needs to be done right now.   A
> have little interest in thoughts and ideas that show no originality.   B
> convey impatience with those who express ideas that are
>   obviously not thought through.   C
> show unintended boredom with talk that is too detailed.   D

Now count up how many As, Bs, Cs and Ds you marked.

Mostly As can be identified as **Realistic** in their style. These people usually place a high value on action and their communication style reflects this. They thrive on getting things done in the here and now and do not like to spend time on what they perceive as unnecessary and time-consuming deliberations. Implementing actions and providing the energy to do this are favourite approaches. They tend to judge others on their actions rather than their intentions and consider it important to exploit the possibilities of each day enthusiastically.

In work they are pragmatic and enjoy the action role and are usually seen by others as wanting to get things done. They can be sought by others who need some drive in a particular situation and whilst they are not usually the instigators of ideas, once they have validated an idea and made sure it will work they wish to get it into play as soon as possible.

Under stress the Realistic will sometimes run the risk of being anti-intellectual by overreacting to differences in opinion and there can be a tendency to ride roughshod over the feelings of others. It is helpful if the Realistic can stand back and view situations with awareness of the feelings and needs of others.

Mostly Bs can be perceived as **Compassionates**. These people place high value on human interaction. They look for contact with others to provide stimulation. They often try to analyse their own emotions and those of others and this can enable them to 'read between the lines'. In a work situation the Compassionate is attracted by jobs that rely on social and interpersonal contacts. They usually have good listening skills and can empathise with the situations of others. They are usually perceived as being dynamic and interesting and have the ability to be aware of the needs of others.

They notice inconsistencies between the speech and actions of people and are sensitive to motives. A good person to have as an orchestrator of interaction between people and to sort out emotional issues. They are also often able to anticipate how others will react to change.

Under stress, the Compassionate can run the risk of being seen as subjective and impulsive. They may take insufficient care with details and be indifferent to some rules. Sometimes their moods can fluctuate widely and they can take things personally and be overreactive, resulting in unnecessary drama and a lack of appropriateness which causes others to question their credibility.

Mostly Cs are the **Considerates**; they place high value on logic, ideas and systematic enquiry. Satisfaction for these people comes from identifying a problem and analysing solutions so that a logical approach can be detected. In a work situation they tend to function in a steady, tenacious manner and do not show emotion. They can be viewed as being sceptical and not willing to proceed with projects until they are satisfied that all the tests have been applied and passed. They are often seen as being consistent producers and logical evaluators of issues and they are valued in organisations for their prudence and analysis rather than their motivation of others.

Under stress a Considerate can be very cautious and rely heavily on his or her style. This can run the risk of being seen as perhaps rigid, overly cautious and averse to risk and sometimes not interested in the feelings of those around them.

Mostly Ds are the **Idealists**. They place high value on ideas, concepts and long-range thinking. They like to spend time considering possibilities and this can be a catalyst for the ideas of people around them. Their style is often challenging as they gain clarity and options from probing and revisiting ideas. In work environments they play active roles in identifying problems, making policies and developing programmes. They are often respected as deep and imaginative thinkers and they tend to question rather than take things for granted. Their ability to project and consider the relationships between things can result in them being described as hard to understand and 'pin down'. They are not overly interested in order and organisation, as they are confident about being able to grasp the implications of things and look at the whole context of areas rather than at particular aspects in isolation.

Under stress, the Idealist runs the risk of being perceived as detached or overly intellectualised and could appear to be indifferent to the reality of the situation. Sometimes they can appear to be inflexible and even impractical and more concerned with the defence of their own ideas rather than putting them into a practical format.

Ways of identifying support

Within large and complex organisations it is almost inevitable that a 'silo' mentality develops where everyone concentrates on the activities and concerns of the particular function or department to which they are assigned. This can create team loyalty but it can also be detrimental to the overall aims of the whole and it certainly makes it more difficult to establish real and productive relationships informally across the organisation as a whole. One of the ways of overcoming the disadvantages of this is to positively build a network of contacts within the organisation who can provide information, support and a continuous widening of influence and sharing of knowledge and skills.

Effective networks contribute towards both interdependence and performance. One very important aspect of responsible decision making is the collection of realistic and valid data. These have to be assimilated before any real analysis or prioritisation can begin. Networking can not only help to ensure your data are appropriate to your problem but can also test the ground about the way that your ideas are likely to be received.

Who to network within the organisation

On a personal basis you can network superiors, peers, subordinates, specialist team members, etc. On a group basis you can network units, departments, divisions, subsidiaries, offices and specialist teams.

How strong is your current knowledge and understanding of the NHS?

- Do you consider that you get to know about the important events, decisions and activities within the organisation?
- Have you maintained your contacts within the organisation as you have moved around?
- Have you kept in touch with operations as you have moved from one department to another?
- Do you regularly read and discuss with others information that comes via the management information systems?
- Do you avoid talking things through face to face, especially pertinent situations and complex problems?
- Do you usually accept or seek the opportunity to make new contacts within the organisation?
- Do you have contacts in a wide range of groups within the organisation or just in your own group?
- Do you actively share information with your peers?
- Do you provide information to your colleagues or are you receptive to others' wishes to discuss organisational matters?
- Have you tried to build up a network for yourself?

- Do you have contact with people in other departments who could help you to acquire information that would enable you to understand and feel part of the future success of the organisation?
- Do you use any source of external information that would add knowledge to your approach?
- Do you gain knowledge and contacts about your line of business from attending trade shows, exhibitions, charitable events, etc.?
- Do you know and talk to your peers in other organisations?
- How well do you manage upwards in your organisation so that situations are easily discussed?
- Do you keep an eye out for pertinent high-level information that could be useful in your work?
- Do you belong to any professional association and take an active part?

In the early days of a career, it is the acquisition of technical skills and knowledge that is vital for progression and professional self-esteem. However, as your career advances, and especially when taking on a management role, although the technical skills do continue to be important you also need the interpersonal skills and understanding to delegate and motivate others. This cannot be achieved overnight and the most successful managers are those who have an action plan that can be flexible but yet provides overall goals to be achieved little by little.

Working in the NHS

Section **Three**

THE ELEMENTS OF COMMUNICATION

OVERVIEW

This section of the book deals with the technical aspects of communication, recognising the fact that communication in the modern health care setting is, thanks to advancing technology, being carried out in a bewildering array of new ways. Despite this the importance of well-developed writing skills must not be lost in the rush to communicate by email, especially as this seems to have a detrimental impact on the use of clear English.

The first chapter in this section, entitled Written Communication, provides a comprehensive and clear overview of how to write clearly and logically. In an era when clinical professionals are being required more and more to explain what they do to an increasingly sceptical public, it seems fair to suggest that high-quality writing will assist greatly in making such matters easy to comprehend. As with many practical skills, there seems neither time nor inclination to teach it in any depth to prequalifying nurses, doctors or other clinical groups. It is for this reason that the decision to include a chapter on this important subject was taken. All too often we assume that we write well although the results rarely bear this out. A cursory perusal of the increasingly impenetrable 'English' contained in many Department of Health circulars and edicts provides further evidence of deficiency. The clear, practical and knowledgeable chapter on writing skills aims to give the reader the necessary insight to improve their skills considerably.

A chapter on the importance of ensuring quality in communication is included. As with the need to write clearly, it is becoming important to know that the key messages of an organisation are understood and that feedback is used to improve services. With the advent of clinical governance in the NHS, the requirements to communicate clearly with the public and use their views to improve services are seen as crucial aspects of improving clinical quality. This chapter discusses how to communicate with stakeholders in the interests of improving the quality of services offered to the public. The chapter is in essence a case study (particularly the application section) from a health-focused organisation that had some serious questions to address with its stakeholders. The lessons learned will be of interest to all readers.

A chapter on information technology was considered to be crucial for any book about understanding communication in the modern health service. The chapter assumes that the reader has no knowledge of the subject thereby ensuring that all aspects of information technology are covered. While some may consider parts of the chapter to be basic, there are still many clinical professionals who privately confess to ignorance of the subject and fear of the technology. In attempting to cater for all levels of knowledge, the chapter aims to be inclusive and comprehensive in the treatment of this important subject.

As with all chapters in the book, application chapters are provided which use case studies, practice checklists or real situations to illustrate key themes.

The elements of communication

Chapter **Eight**

Written communication

Cath Lovatt

OVERVIEW

Writing is a vital tool for communication with each other. As humans, we are unique in the animal kingdom in our use of a written language. But to use this tool effectively does not require a great number of words. Yvonne Bennison of the Industrial Society noted in 1979 that the Ten Commandments consist of only 100 words, the Sermon on The Mount 300 words and the Declaration of Independence 458 words (Isbell 1979).

In contrast, the 1997 White Paper *The new NHS: modern, dependable*, on National Health Service reforms, is over 26 000 words long. Subsequent pronouncements from the Department of Health have been issued on a regular basis in ever denser forms. Whether they convey much sense is open to question.

We are now, therefore, facing an increase in the quantity and form of written materials. We can choose from a whole range of new technologies to transmit messages to each other. Faxes, emails, pager messages and web pages now all compete for our attention with more traditional tools such as newspapers, letters, memos, reports and books. We need the ability to produce simple, accurate and brief written communications if we want to be read and understood clearly.

The key to effective writing is making sure that your reader understands you. It is not just about giving information. Cath Lovatt gives us a clear and detailed overview of written communication with practical examples of how this subject can be approached in the health service. If the government documents of recent years are to be believed, good English and clear written communication seem to be a thing of the past. There is no doubt that we are judged not only by our personal actions but also by what we write. Considering that the written medium is relatively permanent it makes sense to develop a clear, concise and logical writing style. This chapter is included in the book to provide just that – a well-written and easily understood introduction to a skill that seems for many to be a lost (or never acquired) art form.

BARRIERS TO WRITTEN COMMUNICATION

We write because we want a response from the reader. Ineffective writing leads to a breakdown in communication between the writer and the reader. Why should this matter?

In health care, a communication breakdown with readers can cause a range of serious problems. Dissatisfied staff, loss of morale, ill-informed patients, worried relatives, increased complaints, financial loss, bad publicity and wasted time can all result from poor written communication.

This breakdown in communication between the writer and the reader happens because there are barriers which stop the message getting through (Fig. 8.1).

The most common barriers to good written communication result from not thinking about the needs of the reader.

- Message is not clearly structured.
- Message is too long or too complicated to understand.

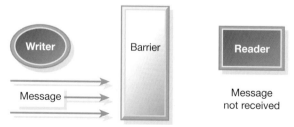

Figure 8.1

The elements of communication

- Message contains jargon words or abbreviations.
- Message uses inappropriate language or grammar.
- Message is of poor quality – badly photocopied, smudged or unclear.
- Message is badly presented with no thought given to layout, design, colour and size of typeface.
- Message is in an inappropriate format – for example, a complex report instead of a brief memo.
- Message is not timely – for example, a report which arrives too late for your manager to act on it.

REMOVING BARRIERS TO EFFECTIVE WRITING

Effective writing is all about understanding your reader and what they need. Before you start writing, consider the following.

- *Who is my reader*? For example, a patient, my manager, clinician, nursing colleagues, the general public.
- *What is my message*? What do I want my reader to do when they have read this?
- *What form of communication should I choose*? For example, letter, memo, email, briefing, report or leaflet.

Who is my reader?

Before you start writing, ask yourself some questions about your intended audience.

- What is their background? Is it the same as mine, e.g. nursing/clinical/patient/general public? Would they use the same language and terminology as me?
- Am I writing to one reader or more than one?
- What do they need to know about me, my department, my organisation?
- What do they already know about this message? Do I need to provide background information?
- What level of detail is required?
- How do they like to receive information?
- When and how will they receive this information? If I want them to do something as a result of this information, will it give them sufficient time to do so?

Written communication

Try to picture your reader as you write. You should take a different approach for different readers, even when writing on the same subject. Professional writers think about their readers. Try the exercise on p. 187 to find out more about how professional journalists write for different types of audiences.

What is my message?

Before you start to write, stop and think about your message. Deciding what you want to say to your audience is the second key step to effective writing. What do you expect your reader to do as a result of reading your words?

For short, simple messages use the journalist's checklist – who? what? why? where? when? and how? This approach ensures that you get the crucial information into your message, without adding unnecessary details. It is particularly suited to letters, memos, emails and press releases.

For longer pieces of writing, try to gather your thoughts into a coherent message by jotting down the key points in any order. Don't worry about finding the right words just yet – it is more important to capture the main issues at the preparatory stage. For each point you can then jot down details as subpoints. For example:

- First key point:
  - first detail
  - second detail
  - third detail
- Second key point:
  - first detail
  - second detail
  - third detail
- Third key point:
  - first detail
  - second detail
  - third detail, etc.

Then you can sort out the order in which you want to present your points, keeping the relevant details with each key point.

What form of communication should I use?

Armed with a good understanding of your reader and a clear idea about your message, you can now decide which form of written communication will be most effective.

Letter

Letters provide a channel of communication between two people and can be used to:

- give or obtain information
- explain or apologise
- create interest
- get action
- record facts.

Use a letter for formal correspondence or for a document that needs to be signed. Don't use a letter if time is important and the matter needs to be resolved as soon as possible.

Try to write it as you would say it, don't suddenly become pompous.

Example: *Every effort is made to adhere to the appointed schedule, however delays can occur due to unanticipated emergency situations.*

Instead: *We will do our best to see you at the time on your clinic card. If there is an emergency then you may have to wait.*

For details on how to lay out a letter, see the example in Application 8.1.

There are several presentation rules to follow which will help to make your letters look modern and professional.

- Don't use commas after each line of the address block.
- Don't use commas for the date – 25 March 2000 not March 25th, 2000.
- Don't use full stops after abbreviated words such as titles. Write Dr or Mrs and not Dr. or Mrs.
- Don't print in a typeface smaller than 12 point – it is too small to be read clearly.

Before you start to write, collect all relevant facts and material together, such as previous correspondence. Check your facts before you start writing. Sort your ideas into a logical sequence and be sure to follow plain English guidelines (see p. 177) as you write.

Memo

Only use a memo (or memorandum) internally within your organisation. Do not send it externally. Use a memo to provide information or to make requests for action but keep it brief. If you need to provide more information you can always attach a separate report.

Whenever you ask for action in a memo, always give a deadline, e.g. *Please let me have your comments by noon on Friday 26 March.*

For details on how to lay out a memo, see the example in Application 8.1.

You can send a memo to more than one recipient at once, e.g.:

To: All practice managers, Westfield Primary Care Group
or
To: All Ward 10 Staff

You can also send a copy of a memo to another recipient for information. This recipient would not be expected to act on the memo; the copy is for information only. Use the initials cc (carbon copy) to denote that the recipient does not need to act on the memo, e.g.:

To: All practice managers, Westfield Primary Care Group
cc: Dr P Smith, Chairman Westfield Primary Care Group

Try not to copy people in on memos unnecessarily. There is a balance between keeping people informed and drowning them in excess paperwork.

You should include job titles in your memo as well as the names of the sender and recipient. People may not know you by name. It also ensures that the memo is understandable in future, even if postholders change.

The same rules about preparing to write a letter also apply to memos. Follow a logical order, using the '5 Ws and H' approach mentioned earlier. Remember to use the active voice – you will make it much easier for your reader to understand what action is required.

Example: *Ward staff are reminded that vehicles must not be parked on the grass verges around the hospital. Failure to comply with this notice will result in cars being clamped and a possible charge being levied for release.*

Prefer: *Please remember – do not park your car on the grass verges around the hospital. The security guard will clamp your car and may charge you to release it.*

Report

A report is simply a tool to present information on a particular topic. You can use it to provide information, to present a case or to give an explanation. Always provide a summary sheet if the report is more than one page long. This allows your reader to understand the key messages without having to wade through pages of detail.

Always use headings to break up the body of the text and to guide your reader through your arguments. The following may be a useful guide to the areas you should cover.

- *Title or title page* – give the name of the report, the organisation, who produced it for whom and when it was written.
- *Summary* – an invaluable overview of the report's findings and recommendations. Try to keep it to between 80 and 120 words.
- *List of contents* – to help the reader find their way around the material. Use wherever you have a report of more than two pages.
- *Introduction or background* – to set the scene as to why the report was produced.
- *Discussion* – develop the arguments or generate alternative solutions.
- *Conclusion* – should follow from the discussion and summarise the main findings.
- *Recommendation* – what should happen as a result of the report?

Minutes and agendas

An agenda is an order of play for a meeting. Sent to invitees in advance of the meeting, it indicates the topics for discussion and who is to lead on each issue. The chairman will use it to guide the team through the issues and to manage time keeping.

Minutes are a record of what was agreed at a meeting. They identify:

- who was present or absent
- any actions to be taken
- who will take each action
- within what timescale.

Minutes follow the order identified in the meeting agenda. They can vary from simple action notes to full verbatim notes of what was said, depending on the type of meeting. Always send minutes to all members, even those who could not attend the meeting. Any errors should be corrected ahead of the next meeting.

Articles

Writing to get published is a time-consuming art, which is a skill in its own right. The same key principles apply to writing for publication as for any other form of written communication:

- know your reader
- be clear about your message
- produce your message in an appropriate format.

Six Steps to **Effective Management**

Albert (1997) advises two different methods of structuring your information. The choice depends on whether you are writing for the academic press or less formal publications.

For the academic press he recommends the IMRD structure.

- *Introduction* – why did we start?
- *Method* – what did we do?
- *Results* – what did we find?
- *Discussion* – what does it all mean?

For all other publications he recommends a BDC structure.

- *Beginning* – used to pull in the reader and set up their interest.
- *Development* – which you should use to take readers through your argument and illustration, step by step.
- *Conclusion* – the message you have already carefully formulated.

Before submitting your work, do check that it is presented in the appropriate style for your target publication.

Briefing

A briefing aims to summarise a complex subject in a short, often single-paged format. It is an effective way to get important information to a selected audience. Briefings are often used as the basis for team cascade meetings, for example, after board meetings or major decisions have been made in an organisation and when the information must be quickly cascaded to all staff.

The person presenting the briefing can pad out the report with details specific to the audience, but the key issues are contained in the briefing note for others who cannot attend the presentation.

You may find this a useful tool for learning sets or departmental meetings, where one member of staff can prepare a briefing for colleagues on a recent journal article or management paper.

Fax

Use a fax when you want to send information quickly and your recipient has stated a preference for a hard copy. Don't use a fax if the message is sensitive or private. Don't send more than a few pages by fax without checking with the recipient – they may prefer you to send the information by other means.

Use a coversheet with your name and details, your recipient's name and details and the total number of pages sent. This way, if the fax fails to transmit properly or is misdirected, your recipient should be able to let you know.

The elements of communication

Use text that is at least 12-point size or it may be difficult to read when it has been transmitted.

If you send a letter by fax, you can type the words 'by fax' on the copy so that both you and your recipient remember that you sent the letter by this method.

Email

Electronic communications are dealt with in detail in Chapter Ten. Use electronic mail for established contacts and less formal mail. Don't use it when you want to present a formal case, especially to your superiors. You naturally tend to use a more relaxed style of writing when using email and because it is so easy to use, it is tempting to be careless. Remember, if you wouldn't put it in a memo, don't put it in an email. Refer to the email checklist in Application 8.1 for more details.

Email saves time in copying and distributing information and probably means that you will get a faster response, if you are sure that your reader has daily access to email. By the nature of health care, many workers do not sit at their computer all day. You may find that other written communication channels offer a better option to get the word out quickly.

Overhead slides and presentation materials

Presentations seem to cause more fear to the uninitiated than any other single area of communications. Presentation skills are covered in Chapter Six. When writing for presentations there are some key pitfalls to avoid, if your moment of glory is to be a success.

Prepare yourself as you would for writing a report or article but don't write your presentation out in full. Plan your presentation materials and write brief speaker's notes, not full pages of text. If you are tempted to write out your text verbatim you will sound wooden when you deliver the presentation. Instead, write a series of key words and bullet points on A4 sheets or index cards to remind you of the themes you want to cover during the talk.

Assuming that you want your audience to read and understand your presentation, be careful when writing for overhead projector or 35 mm slides.

- Don't pack too much onto the slide – your message should fit comfortably onto the front of a T-shirt and still be readable.
- Use a typeface of at least 16 point.
- Use bullet points and key words rather than full lines of text.
- Use pictures, graphs and diagrams to enhance your message.

Written communication

173

Newsletters

The importance of understanding your readers and catering for their various needs is central to writing for a successful newsletter.

Posters and notice boards

A well-maintained notice board can be a simple and effective means of communicating information. A badly maintained board gives negative messages to staff, public and patients about the organisation and misses the opportunity to communicate clearly with your chosen audience.

The Health Services Accreditation Scheme document (1998) on standards to improve the patient's experience suggests that public notice boards must:

- look clean and tidy
- display current notices
- be clearly seen by the public
- indicate any standards for that service
- in outpatients or community clinics, give hours of opening and service phone numbers and the name of the lead clinician and senior nurse on duty
- contain information on how to give feedback on the service or how to make a complaint
- have other information that is relevant to patients or the public; for example, local or national support or self-help groups
- provide information on transport.

When you produce posters for the notice board, don't forget to consider whether people can read the information clearly. The 'what's in it for me?' factor should jump off the page to attract and keep the reader's attention. Small print and cluttered design will not achieve this.

With the increasing availability of desktop publishing and colour printing, it is tempting to go wild with the range of choices. Information can be difficult to read in wacky typefaces, multiple colours or with overuse of illustrations (sometimes known as clip-art). A picture can be worth a thousand words, but only if it helps to give the message impact, not just to fill a gap on the page.

For patients to read information across a waiting room, use A3 or A4 size paper for your poster. The text should be no smaller than 16–20 point. Keep a good colour contrast between the text and the background to improve legibility.

174

The elements of communication

The Royal National Institute for the Blind (1998) recommends black type on white or yellow paper. This is especially important for partially sighted people. Visual impairment is one of the most prevalent age-related disabilities and 67% of the UK's one million registered blind or partially sighted people have one or more additional permanent illnesses or disabilities. The number of NHS consultations is therefore likely to be higher than from the general population for this reason.

Press releases

A press release, or more correctly a 'news release', is information written in a style suitable for use by the media. Health stories are common in the broadcast and print media, reflecting the public appetite for stories with a health angle.

Local media are nearly always interested in human interest stories with a health twist. If you do not have a press officer to help, you may want to write a simple news release to publicise such an event. Stories such as the opening of a new surgery premises, the retirement of a well-known member of staff, the hospital's 10 000th hip operation or a charity walk to raise funds for a new scanner are the type of issues likely to receive positive coverage.

News editors get hundreds of releases each day, so when you write your release, make it easy for the editor to decide quickly whether the story is newsworthy. Use the '5 Ws and H' format to make sure that you include all the necessary details.

- *Who* is the story about?
- *What* happened/will happen?
- *Why* did it happen/is it taking place?
- *Where* did it/will it happen?
- *When* did it/will it take place?
- *How* did it come about?

Put 'News Release' in large type at the top of the page, followed by a date and the title of the release. Make sure that you include a contact telephone number at the bottom of the report in case the reporter needs to talk to you about the story. It is usual to double space the paragraphs so that the editor has space to mark any comments.

Patient information leaflets

Greater emphasis on the involvement and responsibility of patients has been a key theme in recent papers on the future of the

UK's National Health Service. Patients need to have access to appropriate, accurate, relevant and current information about their health. This is central if they are to take responsibility and make informed decisions about their own health and the health of their family.

Patient information leaflets can be one of the most effective and efficient ways to provide written information to patients, especially when used in conjunction with verbal information (Harvey & Plumridge 1991).

Evidently, the quality of the written information is important if the materials are to promote understanding with the intended audience – the patient.

What are the advantages in producing written patient information?

- You can use it to back up verbal information you have given the patient.
- It can give more detail than you can verbally.
- It can help to reassure the patient.
- It can act as a prompt for the patient to ask further questions.
- The patient can keep it for future reference.
- The patient can share it with family and friends.
- You can be sure that each patient gets the same information.

In Application 8.1 there is a checklist for preparing patient information leaflets. However, producing information from start to finish requires a range of skills and you may want to get specialist advice.

You will need to be able to:

- review the current evidence base and present the relative risks of the options
- know how to involve patients and get their feedback on the information
- write in plain language, appropriate to your patient
- understand basic principles of design and layout
- ensure that the format of your information is accessible to all users who need it (e.g. blind or partially sighted patients)
- know enough about printing processes and costs to ensure best value.

The public relations officer, patient liaison officer, the quality department or the library at your local hospital trust or health authority may be able to provide further advice. The Centre for Health Information Quality has excellent information and advice in this area (see Resources).

USING PLAIN ENGLISH

Many people shudder at the memory of trying to learn the rules of grammar in childhood English lessons. So is this what plain English is about?

The first attempt to reform official English was in 1948 with the publication of Sir Ernest Gowers' book, *Plain English*. The theme 'Be short, be simple, be human' was designed to make official forms easier to use. Later, in 1979, the Plain English Campaign presented the idea that layout and design as well as words could influence the effectiveness of a document.

Plain English is not baby language, dumbed-down or oversimplified language. It should not be rude or abrupt. It is not language that puts grammatical correctness before clarity.

Using plain English makes your writing more friendly, direct and easier to understand. The Plain English Campaign suggests that: 'Plain English is writing that gets its meaning across clearly and concisely to its intended audience. It must do this with the necessary impact and the most suitable tone of voice' (1993).

KEY RULES FOR CLEAR WRITING

Keep your sentences short

Get to the point. Use 15–20 words in each sentence. Ninety-five percent of people will understand a sentence of only eight words having read it just once. This figure drops to 4% for a sentence of 27 words (Isbell 1979).

Choose short, familiar words

Don't overcomplicate. Only use jargon if you know that your reader will understand it. Avoid pompous words. Sir Ernest Gowers' *Complete plain words* (1987) contains a useful list of common words and phrases to be used with care.

For example:

> *When we* **commence** *your treatment* . . .
> Prefer: **start** *or* **begin**

> *It is important to* **utilise** *the bed hoist* . . .
> Prefer: **use**

Use commands when writing instructions

Two tablets should be taken with a glass of water . . .
Prefer: *Take two tablets with a glass of water.*

Use the active voice rather than the passive where possible

In the passive voice the 'doer' of the action is either after the verb, as in this example:

The outpatient letter was sent to you by us on the 21 March . . .
Prefer: *We sent you an outpatient letter on 21 March . . .*

or is completely absent. Who is doing the examination here?

It will be necessary for an examination to take place during the appointment . . .
Prefer: *The doctor will examine you during your appointment . . .*

Use the positive rather than the negative where possible

Positive information is much easier to understand.

Visiting is not allowed before 2pm or after 9pm . . .
Prefer: *Visiting hours are between 2pm and 9pm . . .*

Use verbs rather than nouns

Upon arrival please report to the reception desk . . .
Prefer: *When you arrive please report to the reception desk . . .*

Check your spelling

Many word are frequently misspelt. One that regularly appears is *millennium* (it has two n's). There is a useful list of commonly misspelt words in Application 8.1.

Think about punctuation

The humble apostrophe causes many problems, especially *it's* and *its*. Use *it's* as an abbreviation of *it is* only; use *its* to denote possession or ownership.

The elements of communication

178

Check the Further reading section of this chapter for more resources to help you out with basic grammar and punctuation.

Readability

There are several tools to help to assess the relative difficulty of written materials. None of these readability tests is a substitute for writing in plain English to start with. The tools usually measure the number of long words and sentences and relate the results to the reading age necessary to understand the content. In Western industrialised countries like the UK, the average reading age for adults is between 10 and 14 years (Vahabi & Ferris 1995). The Centre for Health Information Quality (1997) reviewed the Flesch and Gobbledygook readability tests.

Flesch

Originally published in 1948 (Flesch 1948), this readability test can be run on many word-processing packages, saving the need to count text manually. However, the results are set against US reading ages rather than UK equivalents. It calculates on four elements: the number of words per sentence; the number of syllables per 100 words; the percentage of personal nouns and pronouns; and the percentage of personal questions or commands. The formula gives two measures of readability with scores between 0 and 100. These are:

- *reading ease*: 0–30 equates with a scientific journal and 90–100 with a comic
- *human interest*: 0–10 equates with a dull scientific paper and 60–100 with a piece of dramatic prose.

Gobbledygook

Ewles & Simnett (1995) calculated this test on two elements: the number of words in a sentence and the number of words with three or more syllables per 100 words. The higher the score, the lower the readability. Tests conducted by the National Consumer Council in 1980 came up with the following results for UK daily newspapers:

- Guardian – 39
- Times – 36

179

- Daily Mail – 31
- The Sun – 26.

There are no software packages capable of performing this test, which has to be undertaken manually.

Gunning-Fog Index

This readability test involves four stages (Secker 1997).

1. Choose a 100-word sample of text from your piece. Count the number of complete sentences in the sample text. Count the total number of words in these sentences. This gives the average sentence length.
2. Count the number of words with three or more syllables in the sample. Numbers and symbols count as less than three syllables and hyphenated words count as two syllables.
3. Add together the average sentence length and the number of words with three or more syllables. Multiply the result by 0.4. This gives you the Fog reading score.
4. Finally, add five to the Fog reading score to get the reading age necessary to understand the written material.

Wright (1999) has examined the limitations of readability indices. She comments that readability indices:

- ignore meaning
- are insensitive to linguistic structure
- overlook how sentences relate to each other
- assume that the material is prose
- do not consider how graphics contribute
- offer no guide for revisions
- may give false assurance.

So although readability tests are useful, they are not enough to ensure that your reader will understand your written communication.

Professional jargon

Why won't health professionals write concise, accessible English? Albert (2000) laments a culture of verbosity and pretension. The NHS seems to have little awareness of how often it fails to communicate in language the general public understands. Its written and spoken communications are all too often incomprehensible (Spiers 1998).

North West Anglia Health Authority set up a group of 150 local people who wanted to learn more about the NHS and held public meetings over 6 months. At the end of that period the health authority found an alarming lack of understanding of terms which the service uses every day and which were used in public consultation documents.

One-third of respondents thought primary care meant life-saving services and more than half thought secondary care meant less urgent services. Sixty-six percent did not know what CPN stood for and 55% did not know what triage was.

Thorogood (1997) argued that scientists use big words and complicated sentences as a way of trying to achieve dominant status. They see it as a question of power rather than of communication. This may be true of other health care professionals too. Different health professions each have their own special jargon which sets them apart. Nurses use different terms from health service planning managers who differ again from surgeons or psychiatrists. This is not an issue until jargon gets in the way, preventing the reader from understanding your message. We need to break down the culture of medi-speak or management-speak and realise that it is OK to use plain English.

How often do you write 'named nurse', 'hospital discharge', 'care plan', 'bed-blocker' or 'primary care' without thinking whether your reader knows what you mean? Jargon is a convenient shorthand in our work. Writing 'coronary artery bypass graft' instead of CABG in the patient's notes every day would not be practical or desirable. However, for a leaflet explaining the operation to a patient, you will need to write a simple explanation, in lay terms, if the patient is to understand fully.

It is a useful exercise to choose some everyday jargon from your specialty and try to give a succinct definition without resorting to more jargon. Try it with a non-medical friend or a relative!

Useful definitions of jargon words which we use frequently in the UK health care setting are available. The Association of Healthcare Communicators (1998) has produced a guide to the structure and operation of the NHS, giving definitions of NHS management-speak. If you don't know what CPN, PCG or HiMP stand for, the *Health Service Journal* has a useful health service acronym buster on its website (see Resources).

Many writers run into problems when writing for a mixed audience. If you have to use jargon for the sake of brevity in a report, then try to include a glossary of terms in an appendix. This way, people unfamiliar with the terms are able to follow your arguments.

Written communication

An obvious example of this occurs in the NHS when health authorities, trusts or primary care groups prepare board papers. Board meetings must be held in public and the papers are often sent to the press and to other members of the local community, who may struggle to appreciate the messages without such an approach.

Presentation

A brief word about presentation. Good writing is not just about the words you use. It is also about how the words appear on the page. Badly laid-out work, with fussy fonts and crammed text are a big turn-off. Make sure you keep a balance of white space on the page. A ragged right margin is easier to read than fully justified text. Size matters. Anything below 12 point is likely to be difficult to read, although this depends on the typeface.

Find out if your organisation has a corporate style for letters, memos and reports. Using this style can help your documents to look professional and corporate.

Once you've produced your work, don't forget that badly photocopied, smudged or unclear writing detracts from your message too.

WEAKNESSES OF WRITTEN COMMUNICATION

There is an apocryphal joke that telepathy and memo are health service managers' preferred methods of communication. In reality, no single method of communication works well in isolation. Make sure that you have a broad range of communication tools at your disposal and know when and how to use them.

There are some shortfalls in using the written word. Marketing communications specialist Wilmshurst (1985) described how 'linear sequential learning theory' can be used to increase the effectiveness of advertising messages. In order for a message to be effective (i.e. result in the desired behaviour), any piece of marketing communication must carry its audience through a series of stages, each dependent on success in the previous stage.

These stages, known as the adoption sequence or AIDA, must first create *awareness* of the issue, commanding the attention of the recipient, which should lead to an *interest*, which once satisfied should make the recipient *desire* the outcome and finally lead to them taking *action* to achieve this.

These stages can also be applied to communication in the health care environment. Ask yourself – what do I want my message to achieve? What do I want the outcome to be? Typical answers might be:

- I want the patient to have a good understanding of their disease, so that they can make an informed decision about their treatment options
- I want my manager to agree to fund my Masters degree course
- I want the complainant to be reassured about the care we gave to their elderly relative
- I want the practice nurses to attend a training day on infection control
- I want the ward staff to fully comprehend the health and safety regulations.

Written communication is not always the best tool to help move the reader between the stages described in the AIDA model. It is very useful for creating awareness (a poster publicising the study day) or for interested people once they need more information (a patient leaflet on treatment choices). It becomes weaker as you move on to stages three and four: creating desire and then action. These are often better reinforced by the power of face-to-face discussions (persuading your manager of your commitment to undertake a further qualification or a difficult meeting with a relative's family) or through group presentations and peer pressure (ensuring that all staff understand health and safety regulations).

In Chapter 2, the theory of communication was explored, including the non-verbal signals we get from body language and voice. With written communication, we lose these additional clues which help us to develop a two-way understanding between people in a face-to-face situation. You do not have the luxury of tailoring your message and the way you deliver it in response to the verbal and non-verbal feedback the recipient gives you.

This puts additional pressure on you as a writer to carefully analyse the reader's position if you are to avoid misunderstandings. If you already know your reader, neurolinguistic programming techniques can help to guide your choice of language so that you tune in to your reader's individual style.

Keep the reader in mind and you should be able to avoid these pitfalls.

CONCLUSION

Carefully researched, simple, accurate and brief writing can be a powerful communication tool. It should aim to be:

Written communication

- *clear* – so that the message is understood by the reader(s)
- *consistent* – so that it supports information coming from other sources. For example, a leaflet given to a patient by the practice nurse should reinforce the verbal advice given by the GP at the surgery
- *cogent* – so that your reader takes the required action because your words are relevant, timely and accurate

and where appropriate

- *corporate* – so that your writing represents the nursing profession, your organisation or the wider NHS in a professional manner.

Practice checklist

- Effective writing is an important management tool. You should aim for writing which can be read and understood by your audience.
- Understanding your reader's needs is central to effective writing. This is particularly important when writing for patients.
- Good writing is brief, simple and clear – avoid jargon, pomposity and complexity.
- Using the right form of writing at the right time increases the effectiveness of your message. Know when to use letters, memos and reports and you will increase your word power.
- Writing is a powerful communication tool when used appropriately. Remember that it also has some inherent weaknesses.

Discussion questions

- Can I explain why effective writing is important and list some common barriers to good written communication in my own workplace?
- Should I be using different forms of communication to increase the effectiveness of my messages?
- Are there any areas of weakness with my own written communication style? What do I need to do to address them?
- What can I do differently today which will improve my written communication?

References

Albert T 1997 Doing the write thing. Health Service Journal 107(5562): 29

Albert T 2000 Getting the wind up. Health Service Journal 110(5699): 30–31

Association of Healthcare Communicators 1998 The NHS route map: a guide to the structure and operation of the NHS. AHC, PO Box 6035, Leighton Buzzard, Bedfordshire LU7 0UD

Centre for Health Information Quality 1997 Quality tools for consumer health information. Topic Bulletin 1. CHIQ, Winchester

Ewles L, Simnett I 1995 Promoting health: a practical guide, 3rd edn. Scutari, London, pp 263–264

Flesch R 1948 A new readability yardstick. Journal of Applied Psychology 32(3): 221–233

Gowers E (revised Greenbaum S, Whitcut J) 1987 The complete plain words, 3rd edn. Penguin, London

Harvey JL, Plumridge RJ 1991 Comparative attitudes to verbal and written medical information among hospital outpatients. Annals of Pharmacotherapy 25: 925–928

Health Services Accreditation Scheme 1998 Focus on patients: standards to improve the patient's experience. Health Services Accreditation, Battle, East Sussex

Isbell P 1979 A guide to letter writing. The Industrial Society, London

Plain English Campaign 1993 The Plain English story. PO Box 3, New Mills, High Peak SK22 4QP

RNIB 1998 See it Right Campaign. RNIB, 224 Great Portland Street, London W1N 6AA

Secker J 1997 Assessing the quality of patient-education leaflets. Coronary Health Care 1: 37–41

Spiers H 1998 Clarity begins at home. Health Service Journal 108(5594): 28–30

Thorogood N 1997 Questioning science: how knowledge is socially constructed. British Dental Journal 183: 152–155

Vahabi M, Ferris L 1995 Improving written patient education materials: a review of the evidence. Health Education Journal 54: 99–106

Wilmshurst J 1985 The fundamentals of advertising. Heinemann, London

Wright P 1999 Readability index: life-line or weak link? Hi Quality Matters 5: 1–2

Further reading

Burchfield RW (ed) 1996 The new Fowler's modern English. Oxford University Press, Oxford

Chapman J, Langridge J 1997 Physiotherapy health education literature. Physiotherapy 83(8): 406–411

Gregory W 1996 The informability manual. Making information more accessible in the light of the Disability Discrimination Act. HMSO, London

Six Steps to **Effective Management**

Plain English Campaign 1994 Utter drivel. A decade of jargon and gobbledygook. Robson Books, London

Short Words. A twice-yearly newsletter on effective written communications. Tim Albert Training, Dorking. www.timalbert.co.uk

Resources

http://www.plainenglish.co.uk
This is the home of the UK's Campaign for Plain English. It has a useful on-line guide to writing letters, with exercises to test your new-found skills.

http://www.plainlanguage.gov
This excellent site helps you to create user-friendly documents. PLAN (Plain Language Action Network) is a US government-wide group which aims to improve communications with the public.

http://webster.commnet.edu/ HP/pages/darling/original.htm
If you are interested in learning more details about writing and grammar, this US-based site is excellent. It is entirely free of charge and you can test yourself with some comprehensive grammar exercises and quizzes. However, don't forget that some US spellings differ from those in the UK.

http://www.leeds.gov/lcc/equalops/eq _ home.html
The Equal Opportunities Unit at Leeds City Council has produced several useful guidelines on using plain English.

http://www.hfht.org/chiq
Centre for Health Information Quality (CHIQ) provides a regular newsletter and research on this eponymous topic. Highcroft, Romsey Road, Winchester, Hants SO22 5DH. Tel 01962 863511 ext.200.

http://www.discern.org.uk
DISCERN is a general set of quality criteria for the content of written health information on treatment choices.

http://www.hsj.co.uk
The *Health Service Journal* site offers a toolbox section with a variety of 'How to..' materials, excellent if you are new to health service management. It also has an NHS jargon buster. Access is free to most areas of the site, but you will need to register by supplying some basic details and choosing a password. Journal subscribers can also review archive material.

Application **8:1**

Cath Lovatt

Practical exercises to test your writing skills

INTRODUCTION

This chapter contains a series of exercises, worked examples and checklists to help you improve your writing skills. They are drawn from a variety of sources, including the NHS, and reflect real written communications management challenges for nurses.

TAILORING THE MESSAGE

Try this practical exercise to examine how professional journalists write. (You may prefer to do this as a group exercise with colleagues.)

Identify a current health issue as the story breaks in the press. Health stories happen fairly frequently as health is always news. Typical examples include stories about the latest clinical breakthrough, nursing shortages or a funding dilemma for the NHS.

Get copies of the coverage in national daily newspapers. In the UK you might choose the *Guardian*, the *Daily Telegraph*, the *Daily Mail* and the *Sun*. If you have one, you should also get a copy of your local regional daily newspaper. Don't forget to look at the editorial comment as well as news stories and features.

Now take a look at how the professional press cover the same story. Visit your local medical library and look at publications such as *Nursing Times*, the *Health Service Journal*, *Doctor* and *GP Magazine* or the news pages of the *British Medical Journal*. If you cannot obtain copies of the papers and journals, you could take a look at the news pages of their websites instead.

Compare how the different print media cover your chosen issue. Discuss the differences in style, language and message.

The nursing press will use a different approach from the medical press but they will probably both use clinical jargon and abbreviations that you will not see in national broadsheets or in the tabloids.

Local newspapers tend to write from their regional perspective. They try to illustrate the issue to people in their area, using case studies with links to the story. For example, imagine a story about a patient awaiting her heart transplant in Newcastle. Regional press coverage might contain comments from a local patient who has already had the operation.

Notice how professional writers tailor the content and style of writing to suit their readers, even when covering similar issues. Try to tailor what you write to match your audience, by thinking about what your reader needs and wants.

CHOOSING YOUR TOOL

Make a list of some situations in your own area of work where written communication is necessary. For example:

- reply to a letter of complaint
- plans to allocate winter beds
- date of a leaving do for a colleague
- initiating a discussion
- making a proposal for changes in the ward shift pattern.

Decide who your reader is and which method of written communication is most suitable for the task. Does the situation warrant a report, letter, memo, email or briefing note? Some examples are set out in Table 8.1.1.

USING A READABILITY TEST

Find a piece of your written work which is at least 200–300 words long. You could use a letter, a memo, a patient leaflet, a review article or a report. If you haven't written anything recently, find a leaflet or a newspaper article written by somebody else.

For whom do you think the material was written? Was it for fellow nurses, for your manager, for patients, for the general public or perhaps for children? Do you think it contains any language or jargon which the intended reader would not understand?

Using the instructions on page 180 for the Gunning-Fog Readability Index, work out the reading age required to understand the piece. Does the reading age match the intended

Table 8.1.1 Examples of some typical messages and the audiences at which they are aimed. Suggested forms of writing are given

Message	Reader	Form of writing
Query about overspend on the ward budget for surgery	Management accountant	Memo or email
Introduction of a new policy for nurses' uniforms	Trust Board	Report
Advice about treatment options for back pain	Patient	Leaflet
Information about how to refer patients to the new consultant surgeon	General practitioners	Letter
Confirmation of pay settlement	All nursing staff	Briefing note followed by personal letter
Additional copy of map and road directions to tomorrow's training day	Speaker travelling from another town	Fax or email

audience? If not, what steps could you take to simplify the writing?

Hints:

- use shorter sentences
- avoid jargon – use simple language
- use the active voice rather than the passive.

WRITING PATIENT INFORMATION

This exercise will help you to practise many of the skills needed for writing in a health care setting. You are going to draft an information leaflet for patients visiting your clinic or surgery for the first time. Imagine that your patient has never been to your hospital, clinic or surgery before.

Think about your audience. What do they already know and what do they need to know? How can you present the information as clearly as possible? What sort of language should you use? Are there any jargon terms you should avoid or explain?

They will need to know where to go and what to expect on the day. Do they need to bring anything with them? Will they undergo any investigations? What are the side effects? Who will they see? How long will it take? Is it safe to drive afterwards?

Six Steps to **Effective Management**

Make sure that you think about:

- the structure of your information
- your choice of language
- how you present the information
- the evidence base for any clinical information.

If possible, ask some patients for their opinions of the draft and amend the leaflet to include their feedback.

When you have finished, use the checklist in Box 8.1.1 to see if you missed any important issues.

How did you do? If you ticked most of the areas – well done. You now have a set of skills which are essential to understanding and producing good written communication. If not, go back and analyse where you need to do some more work. Plan how you will develop the necessary knowledge and skills.

PATIENT INFORMATION CHECKLIST

Patient information is one of the most important areas to get right. Secker (1997) has produced a very useful checklist for assessing the quality of patient information leaflets.

Box 8.1.1 Checklist for patient information leaflets (after Secker (1997) © Harcourt Health Sciences, with permission)	
Information	Up to date and accurate
	No unnecessary detail
	Order reflects patients' priorities
	Well organised under section headings
Headings	Relevant to patients (action oriented or question and answer)
	Stand out from the main body of the text
	Aligned with the main body of the text (not centred)
Writing style	Reading age no higher than 10 or 11 years
	Personalised, everyday language
	Language inclusive and respectful of individuality
Colour	Attractive
	Not intrusive
Text design	Clear, uncluttered font
	12-point type or larger
Illustrations	Simple and uncluttered
	Meaningful to patients
	Positioned close to relevant text
	Inclusive and acceptable

Use the checklist in Box 8.1.1 to make sure that the key areas are covered. You can use this to assess your own design or to critically evaluate an existing leaflet. It can be helpful to do this exercise in a group.

I would also add the question: Have patients been involved in the design and writing of this leaflet? This need not be done in a very formal way. For example, you might ask some patients to look over a leaflet and let you know what they think while they are waiting for a review appointment.

EMAIL

Email is a new form of written communication which breaks down many traditional rules of etiquette. Here are some email do's and don'ts (after Hull & East Riding Community NHS Trust 1999, with permission).

Do

- Keep messages short and use a meaningful title.
- Only send to relevant people and avoid unnecessary copies to others.
- Be polite – recipients appreciate the use of first names.
- Use distribution lists sensibly and understand who they include.
- Think about the content and style of the document. Your recipient may not be able to view pictures, graphs or logos or open your attachments.
- Inform the helpdesk if you receive anything of an illegal nature (e.g. racist or pornographic material).

Don't

- Include all recipients when replying, unless it is relevant to them.
- Send angry emails. If replying to one that made your blood boil, answer it later when you've calmed down.
- Include things others should not see. Forwarded emails can be embarrassing for the originator (you!).
- Include defamatory or untrue statements in emails (an insurance company was sued for libel and had to pay thousands of pounds in damages).
- Send racist or sexist remarks in emails or attach illegal documents (employers have sacked employees for this).

Practical exercises to test your writing skills

COMMONLY MISUSED WORDS

Use this list to check your knowledge of some words which are often confused. Make a note of any which you think you need to remember. Consider buying a dictionary of English usage if you are still unsure.

accept to take, acknowledge (*I accept your criticism.*)
except to exclude, excluding (*Visiting hours are 10–7 daily, except Sundays.*)

affect to produce a change or alteration (*Drinking can affect your health.*)
effect to bring about, accomplish (*The physiotherapy effected an immediate improvement in the patient's mobility.*)

aural of hearing (*The nurse arranged an aural examination for the patient.*)
oral spoken; concerning the mouth (*The manager gave oral approval to proceed, but confirmed the arrangements in writing.*)

complement to suit, complete (*That colour complements your eyes nicely.*)
compliment to praise (*She complimented the nurse on her sterile technique.*)

diagnosis identification of a condition or problem (*My diagnosis of the patient's condition is Menière's disease.*)
prognosis forecast (*His prognosis is poor as he has reduced lung function.*)

stationary not moving (*The trolley was stationary in the corridor.*)
stationery paper goods (*There was no paper in the office stationery cupboard.*)

disinterested not involved, impartial (*A disinterested observer at the meeting would not have understood the medical jargon.*)
uninterested not interested, indifferent (*The chief executive was uninterested in the consultants' reaction to her decision.*)

(adapted from *The Hutchinson Almanac* 2001, © Helicon Publishing Limited 2000, with permission)

The elements of communication

COMMONLY MISSPELT WORDS

Do you have problems with any of the words in Box 8.1.2? Make a note of any which you are unsure about and keep it handy when you write.

Box 8.1.2 Commonly misspelt words (*Hutchinson Almanac* 2001, © Helicon Publishing Limited 2000, all rights reserved)

accommodation	exercise	occurrence
achieve	exhilarate	omit
address	extravagant	oneself
aggressive	February	parallel
amount	foreign	paraphernalia
appearance	friend	permissible
asphalt	fulfil	personnel
attach	gauge	poisonous
banister	government	possess
beautiful	grammar	potatoes
beginning	guarantee	practice (noun)
budgeted	guard	practise (verb)
business	harass	precede
cemetery	height	prejudice
cigarette	hygiene	privilege
collapsible	hypocrisy	profession
committee	idiosyncrasy	pronunciation
competition	immediately	publicly
conscientious	independent	questionnaire
controversial	(noun and adjec-	receive
definitely	tive)	repellent
dependant (noun)	install	separate
dependent (adjec-	instalment	sergeant
tive)	jewellery	siege
describe	league	sieve
desiccate	liaise	sincerely
desperate	library	soldier
detach	literature	solemn
diarrhoea	manoeuvre	supersede
diphtheria	Mediterranean	targeted
disappear	millennium	terrestrial
disappoint	millionaire	tomatoes
dissect	mischievous	tranquillity
dissipated	mortgage	traveller
ecstasy	necessary	unnecessary
eighth	neither	until
embarrass	niece	unusual
exaggerate	noticeable	unwiedly
excellent	nuisance	vetoed
excitement	occasion	videoed

Practical exercises to test your writing skills

WORKED EXAMPLES OF DOCUMENTATION

Sample layouts for the most widely used forms of written communication – the memo and the letter – are given in Figures 8.1.1 and 8.1.2, respectively

Always ask if your organisation has a house style. If there is one, use it. A readily identifiable style helps to increase professionalism and a sense of corporacy, amongst both staff and the public. This in turn helps to communicate your message.

PLAIN ENGLISH – BEFORE AND AFTER EXAMPLES

The translations in Box 8.1.3 are reproduced with permission from the Plain English Campaign. Notice how much shorter and clearer they are than the original versions. Have a go at rewriting one of the paragraphs for yourself, before you look at the Plain English translation.

> **Box 8.1.3** Plain English translations (from the Plain English Campaign, with permission)
>
> **Before**: 'High-quality learning environments are a necessary precondition for facilitation and enhancement of the ongoing learning process.'
>
> **After**: 'Children need good schools if they are to learn properly.'
>
> **Before**: 'If there are any points on which you require explanation of further particulars we shall be glad to furnish such additional details as may be required by telephone.'
>
> **After**: 'If you have any questions, please ring.'
>
> **Before**: 'It is important that you shall read the notes, advice and information detailed opposite then complete the form overleaf (all sections) prior to its immediate return to the Council by way of the envelope provided.'
>
> **After**: 'Please read the notes opposite before you fill in the form. Then send it back to us as soon as possible in the envelope provided.'
>
> **Before**: 'Your enquiry about the use of the entrance area at the library for the purpose of displaying posters about the provenance and authoritativeness of the material to be displayed.
>
> Posters and leaflets issued by the Central Office of Information, the Department of Health and Social Security and other authoritative

> *(cont.)*
> bodies are usually displayed in libraries, but items of a disputatious or polemic kind, whilst not necessarily excluded, are considered individually.'
>
> **After**: 'Thank you for your letter asking permission to put up posters in the entrance of the library.
>
> Before we can give you an answer we will need to see a copy of the posters to make sure they won't offend anyone.'

The Department of Health won a Plain English Campaign award in December 1999 for a leaflet intended to cut overuse of antibiotics (Fig. 8.1.3). 'Antibiotics – don't wear me out' was described as an 'effective tool at getting information across' and commended for its use of cartoon character Andy Biotic, 'a no-nonsense antibiotic capsule'. It explains to patients that antibiotics work only against bacterial infections and not against the common cold viruses.

Contrast this clearly communicated message with winner of the Plain English Campaign's 1999 Golden Bull Award. Golden Bull Awards are given for the year's worst example of gobbledygook. The award takes into account how bad the documents are and how they affect the lives of ordinary people. It was presented to a hospital in Scotland for a patient information card (Fig. 8.1.4).

References

Hull and East Riding Community NHS Trust 1999 Some e-mail do's and dont's. H&ERCNT, Hull

Hutchinson Almanac 2001. Helicon Publishing Limited 2000, Oxford (www.helicon.co.uk)

NHS Executive Communications Unit 2000 Templates for letterhead, fax and memo in NHS corporate style in: NHS identity guidelines (draft). NHS Executive, DoH

Plain English Campaign DoH

Secker J 1997 Assessing the quality of patient-education leaflets. Coronary Health Care 1: 37–41

Resources

Plain English Campaign website: http://www.plainenglish.co.uk

Practical exercises to test your writing skills

INTERNAL MEMO ST. ANYWHERE NHS TRUST

From: A Sender, Surgical Nurse Manager   Ext: 3078

To: See distribution list

cc: C Jones, Superintendent Physiotherapist

Date: 20 June 2000   Ref: AS/tt

Subject: **How To Set Out A Memo**

At our team meeting last Wednesday (18 June 2000) some of the F grade staff asked me for advice on setting out a memo. This memo layout should help. Always ask if there is a corporate style before setting out your own.

Use memos to give a message or propose an action. The main points for the address section above are:

- Use job titles as well as names.
- Don't use punctuation in the date or in forms of address.
- Use your initials and the typist's initials as a reference (optional).
- If there is more than one addressee, you can use a distribution list at the base of the memo to list the names and job titles.
- 'cc' means carbon copy and is used to indicate a copy for information, not for action.

The main points for the body of the memo are:

- Use a ragged right margin and a minimum 12 point typeface for increased legibility.
- Get to the point.
- Be concise and use simple direct language.
- Use the active voice.
- Give a deadline for any action.

Please sign and return your training record forms to me by 26 June.

A Sender

Surgical Nurse Manager

Distribution:

A Smith, F Grade nurse
L Green, Manager Ward 10
C Brown, Ward 10 Clerk

Figure 8.1.1   How to set out an internal memo (from NHS Executive Communications Unit 2000, with permission).

The elements of communication

Bigtown, Midvale and Smallwick

NHS Trust

Your reference: ABC/JJ

Our reference: 2000/01/AS

Contact: Miss A Sender, direct dial 623078

Bigtown Hospital
1 Fiction Road
Countytown
Anyshire
L12 3AB

Tel: 01234 567 890
Fax: 01234 098 765

Mr J Fowler
21 Chestnut Ave
Bigtown
Westshire
BT3 5HP

16 July 2000

Dear Mr Fowler

Re Advice About Writing Letters

Thank you for your letter asking me how to set out a letter. Check whether your organisation has a corporate style for letters. If there is one - use it. If not, this is what I recommend.

- Type the references and the name and address of the person you are writing aligned to the left. Make sure that their address details will show if you use a window envelope.

- Use a plain typeface like Arial or Times New Roman at a minimum of 12 point size.

- If your writing comes within 20mm of the bottom of the page, continue on another page. Make sure that there are at least three lines, except for your signature on the second page.

- Leave at least five or six lines after 'Yours sincerely' for the signature.

I hope that this answers your questions. Please ring me if you need more information.

Yours sincerely

Alice Sender
Nurse Manager

Figure 8.1.2 Letter layout (from NHS Executive Communications Unit 2000, with permission).

Practical exercises to test your writing skills

The elements of communication

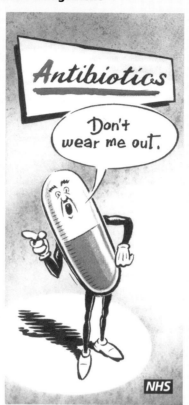

Figure 8.1.3 Plain English award-winning leaflet 'Don't wear me out' puts across a complex message in plain language (with permission from DoH).

> YOU HAVE HAD AN INTRA-ARTICULAR INJECTION OF STEROID
>
> *Facial flushing a few days after the injection is normal, however in the event of increasing pain, swelling or redness of the joint, urgent assessment is mandatory. Aspiration of joint fluid with appropriate culture may be necessary.*

Figure 8.1.4 This patient information card won the 1999 Plain English Campaign Golden Bull Award (with permission from the Plain English Compaign).

Example of a patient information leaflet: The Royal Marsden

The text that follows is taken from a patient information leaflet produced by The Royal Marsden NHS Trust (with permission).

CARE OF A SKIN-TUNNELLED CATHETER

What is a skin-tunnelled catheter?

A skin-tunnelled catheter is a tube which is inserted through your chest into a large vein leading to your heart.

The catheter is made of a non-irritant material such as silicone, which means it can be left in place for several weeks or months. Along the catheter, there is a small cuff which you may be able to feel through your skin. This cuff prevents the catheter from moving or falling out.

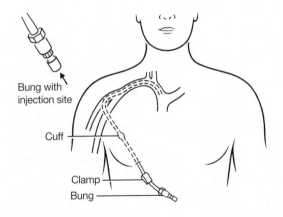

The catheter can be used to give fluids and drugs. It may also be possible to take blood samples from it. The catheter will save you, or your child, from having repeated needle pricks during treatment. The catheter may contain two or more tubes in one – this is called a **double-lumen** or **multi-lumen** catheter.

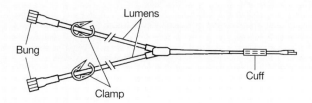

Along each lumen is a **clamp** which opens and closes the catheter. It is used to prevent leakage.

At the end of each lumen is a cap called a **bung**. This protects the catheter and also prevents leakage.

How is the catheter inserted?

A doctor will insert the catheter, usually using a local anaesthetic which numbs an area on your chest. You will also be given a mild sedative to relax you and make you sleepy. Occasionally a general anaesthetic may be used.

Only two small cuts will be made on your chest, one to tunnel the catheter and the other, near the collar bone, to insert it into your vein. You will have two stitches, one at each site. You will be told when these should be removed and by whom.

A chest x-ray will be done to check the catheter is in the right place.

During insertion the guidewire may scratch the top of your lung and cause a **pneumothorax** (air pocket). This could make you slightly breathless but it would show up on the x-ray and be treated straight away.

Who will look after the catheter?

At first the nurses will look after the catheter then they will teach you how to care for it. Before you go home, you should have had plenty of practice and as much teaching as you need.

Care of the catheter

We will give you the following articles to take home:

1. Some spare bungs
2. A spare clamp
3. A supply of Hepsal ampoules 50 i.u. in 5 ml
4. Some needles and syringes
5. A supply of spirit swabs to clean the injection site on the bung
6. Some sterile gauze and tape, if you have been told to keep the catheter site covered or wish to do so
7. A container to dispose of sharp items.

If you have any problems at home, please don't hesitate to ring the ward where you (or your child) were last an inpatient or ask to be connected with the intravenous team, chemotherapy nurse, or doctor (see the back of this leaflet).

The three important points to remember are:

● you must always wash your hands before handling your catheter
● your catheter must be kept clean at the exit site, where it comes out of your chest
● you must flush your catheter once a week to keep it clear, using 5 ml (50 i.u.) of Hepsal.*

*Local practices may vary.

To keep the catheter clear

1. Gather together all the articles you need on a clean surface.
2. Wash your hands well, and dry them.
3. Fit a green needle on to the end of a syringe.
4. Break the Hepsal ampoule as instructed.
5. Draw up the Hepsal.
6. Change the needle on the syringe to a blue one.
7. Wipe the bung with a spirit swab and wait for it to dry.
8. Insert the needle through the injection point and open the clamp.
9. Slowly inject the contents of the syringe.
10. Keep your thumb on the plunger of the syringe and close the clamp on the catheter.
11. Remove the needle and syringe and place them and the ampoule into the container you have been given.

If you have a multi-lumen catheter you must inject all tubes in the same way, using a new set of equipment each time.

Example of a patient information leaflet

Six Steps to **Effective Management**

Special advice and teaching will be given if you are receiving drugs continuously using a small infusion pump. You may also be given another booklet in this series *Ambulatory Chemotherapy* (No. 34).

Remember:

Every four weeks you need to change the bung. You should do this before you flush your catheter.

a. Gather together all the articles you need on a clean surface.
b. Wash your hands well and dry them.
c. Check that the clamp on the catheter is closed.
d. Remove the bung and throw it away.
e. Put a new bung on the end of the catheter.
f. Go through the procedure of clearing the catheter as before (1–11).

Care of the exit site

You (or your child) should have a bath, shower or all over wash every day to keep your skin generally clean. You don't need to use antiseptics.

Don't immerse your body totally in the bath so that the exit site or catheter is under the water. After your bath use a fresh bowl of ordinary warm tap water and cotton wool to wash and dry around the catheter. Don't use the same water, cloth or towel that you've used for the rest of your body.

Following a shower pat the area dry with cotton wool. After a bath, shower or wash gently wipe once around the exit site with a spirit swab and allow the skin to dry.

Tape the catheter to your skin so it doesn't pull at the exit site. Put a dry gauze dressing over the site, if you wish to, and tape it in position. You must change this dressing every day.

Contact the hospital immediately if any of the following occur:

- You experience cold, shivery, flu-like symptoms
- There is any swelling, redness or discharge at the catheter exit site
- You have any chest pain or pain in your arm or neck
- There are signs of swelling of your arm or neck

Removal of the catheter

When your catheter is due to be removed you will be admitted to hospital, usually as a day patient. A blood test may be done when you arrive to check if your blood count is satisfactory.

Local anaesthetic will be injected into the area around the cuff and then a small cut will be made. The cuff will be removed, along with the catheter. Two or three stitches are used to close the cut and a dressing will be applied. The procedure takes about 30–60 minutes.

The hole in your vein closes up naturally within about half an hour. You will be asked to rest flat on the bed for a while before you can go home. The stitches can be removed a week later by your family doctor (GP) or district nurse.

If anything unusual occurs and you are worried, don't hesitate to telephone:

Your ward . . . .

or your hospital doctor . . . .

or your chemotherapy nurse . . . .

at . . . . Hospital

Telephone number . . . .

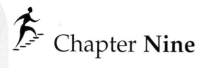

Chapter **Nine**

Quality communication

Stuart Skyte

- **Customers and stakeholders**
- **Customer perceptions of quality**
- **Customer satisfaction surveys**
- **National initiatives**

O V E R V I E W

In this chapter Stuart Skyte discusses the important aspect of quality in communication. The health services are constantly reminded of the need to communicate with patients or customers more readily than has been the case previously. Although the commercial health care sector has a lot of experience in this field the NHS is having to catch up quickly. It was therefore deemed important to include a chapter such as this to give clinical professionals an appreciation of some of the techniques used in communicating with patients and carers, or stakeholders as they have become known in recent years. The chapter provides useful insight into exactly who these people might be.

Bound up within the huge subject of quality is the perception of what a health care organisation does or how the service it offers might be thought of. Stuart Skyte gives some lively examples of how quality is perceived along with practical thoughts on solutions. This is very topical and the chapter reminds us that we need to work hard not only to improve quality in the real sense but to inform our stakeholders of this. Similarly, engaging them in the process is a concept many health professionals struggle with, though it does not have to be threatening. This is where the link with communication comes into play.

Finally the author declares that he works for the United Kingdom Council for Nursing, Midwifery and Health Visiting (UKCC). This body, now the Nursing and Midwifery Council, has steadily improved the quality of its communication to the public and the three professions it regulates. He relates how a large survey (described in detail in Application 9.1) assisted the council in its efforts to improve its image and work. There are some useful pointers for the health services, especially with links to clinical governance and the NHS Plan being made clear. This chapter adds some of the points made by Cath Lovatt to round out the book very well.

INTRODUCTION

The purpose of this chapter is to put all the skills and techniques learned in previous chapters into a wider context, namely that successful communications are based on knowing and satisfying customer needs. There would, for example, be little point in devising a brilliant advertising campaign for a product that nobody wants because it doesn't work. By appreciating the fact that patients and clients are actually the customers of health and social care providers and that, as such, their needs and wants should lie at the heart of that provision, communications become more focused and fruitful. Ultimately, smart communications is telling people what you have already established they want to hear because that is what they actually want from their health care.

CUSTOMERS AND STAKEHOLDERS

Customers are always stakeholders but stakeholders are not always customers. That sounds like a riddle but it is a truism. A customer is someone who purchases or uses your products or services. In the commercial world, getting a product from the manufacturer to the person who buys it in the shop is a process involving many customers, only some of whom are shown below.

Raw materials providers ⎫
Machine tool providers ⎬ → Manufacturers → Wholesalers →
Energy providers   ⎭   Retailers → Purchasers

Quality communication

While there may be many in the chain, the relationships are straight-forward. Are there the same relationships in the public sector generally and the health services specifically? There is evidence that rail passengers resent the way in which they have been reclassified by the railway companies as customers but that is what they are. In fact, they are both. They don't cease to be passengers when they are treated as customers. By thinking of patients and clients as customers, it helps you to focus on them and their needs.

Who are your customers?

Traditionally, the health care professional has always been right but now the customer is right ... at the heart of the NHS. The National Plan, published in July 2000, makes that abundantly clear. In her response to the Plan, quoted in the *Nursing Times* (27 July 2000), Karlene Davis, General Secretary of the Royal College of Midwives, said: 'This is a huge cultural change. We shouldn't be afraid to call service users customers'. The section on national initiatives (p. 216) goes into more detail about the National Plan.

Karlene Davis is right but it is extraordinary that patients and clients have had to wait more than 50 years in order to be treated as customers in the NHS. No organisation, whether in the private or public sector, can realistically ignore the needs and wants of its customers and be truly successful. In the NHS, customer awareness has been largely ignored while the needs of the system have tended to be put first. Why is that?

Business orientations

All businesses have orientations and four distinct types have been identified: customer orientation; marketing orientation; production orientation; and system orientation. What typifies these different orientations, does the way an organisation communicates reflect its overriding orientation and are you able to identify your own organisation from the following descriptions?

In a *customer-oriented* organisation – perhaps a traditional corner shop – staff are responsive to the individual needs of the customers, however specific, unusual and difficult to fulfil; they have a customer focus. The customer is king and the business is maintained on the basis of repeat customers. Could a hospital or clinic be run along these lines? Its communications would reflect openness, accessibility and giving the patients what they want when they want it.

In a *marketing-oriented* organisation – perhaps a PR or advertising agency – there is constant striving to establish what the customers want and how this can be delivered. There is an emphasis on customer feedback and market research (see section on customer satisfaction surveys, p. 212). Are such organisations necessarily small and, if so, could a small clinic or GP practice be so orientated? Could larger health provider organisations adopt this marketing approach?

In a *production-oriented* organisation – typically a manufacturing company – everybody is geared to getting the product just right from the company's point of view, even if it may not be absolutely perfect for the customer and the delivery date and after-sales service may be inadequate. There is an engineering focus and people are fascinated by the product rather than the customer.

In a *systems-oriented* organisation – NHS hospitals are perfect examples of this – the system rules. There are standard procedures, rules and forms for everything, there is little scope for individuality, the hierarchy is rigid and the customer is barely considered. Do public sector organisations have to be like this? Who benefits from these behaviours? Does, for example, the way that hospital appointments are made and communicated reflect this?

Who are your stakeholders?

The NHS is starting to recognise that patients and clients are their customers but who and what are their stakeholders? If you live next door to a GP practice, you are a stakeholder whether or not you are on the patient list. If your spouse is undergoing hospital treatment, you aren't a customer but you are a stakeholder. If the UKCC removes a nurse from the register for professional misconduct and you are a nurse, the surrounding publicity may affect you as a stakeholder. If you are a tax payer, you are a stakeholder in every public service.

We are all multiple stakeholders in a vast number of enterprises. A stakeholder can be defined as someone who has a direct or indirect interest in an organisation or company. Mitroff (1983) defined stakeholders as people who have a vested interest in an enterprise, those who are influenced by or who influence it. For example, the UKCC's stakeholders include:

- those on its register, namely nurses, midwives and health visitors
- employers of nurses, midwives and health visitors

- the professional bodies and trades unions which represent nurses, midwives and health visitors
- consumers (embracing patients, clients, carers, the general public)
- government and Parliament
- its staff and former staff
- other regulatory bodies in the UK and around the world
- its suppliers
- its neighbours in Portland Place
- the four National Boards.

There is a difference between customers and stakeholders, but does it matter? Is it an artificial distinction? It is important to distinguish between the two as you communicate with them about different things. Communication with customers is more narrowly focused. For example, a health centre's communications with its customers might be about a change in its opening hours, new services provided at the centre, new parking arrangements, new staff or a new appointments system. These would only affect its customers at the point when they want treatment or advice. Communications with its stakeholders could be more broad based and not confined to a specific point of contact. For example, the health centre might be considering a change of status which, while not directly affecting its patients, would be of interest to stakeholders such as the health authority, the Community Health Council, the local MP and local NHS trusts as well as its patients.

Communicating with stakeholders is often about involvement in and consultation about the organisation – how the 'business' is run, new ideas, governance, longer term strategy. As such, the style of the communication has to be more open, a more listening approach. Organisations therefore often use media such as consultative conferences and workshops, focus groups and one-to-one meetings to communicate with their stakeholders. It is also important to maintain regular contact with your key stakeholders, perhaps via regular briefings and newsletters, but they should not be overwhelmed with trivia and detail. If you have been treated in a hospital (a customer), on the other hand, the last thing you want are constant communications from that hospital about all manner of developments, which would only serve to remind you of what may have been an unpleasant episode in your life.

For communications purposes, you do have to differentiate between customers and stakeholders. In a crude sense, your customers are people you do business with but your stakeholders are your longer term friends.

The elements of communication

CUSTOMER PERCEPTIONS OF QUALITY

The advent of Total Quality Management (TQM) in the 1990s was essentially about thinking of quality in a much broader way than hitherto, traditionally quality control at the end of the production line. TQM is a way of achieving customer orientation within an organisation by encouraging everyone who provides a service – and that must mean every employee – to adopt a customer perspective on what they do. TQM is not just another ephemeral management tool which quickly passes into misuse as the next one emerges from the Harvard Business School. Morgan & Murgatroyd (1994) argue that it is a deeply ingrained philosophy, an organisational ethic, designed to satisfy the needs of all customers within an organisation, both internal and external. Unhappily, and perhaps unfairly, they also argue that there are problems in trying to inculcate TQM into public sector organisations. But what is quality, particularly within the context of the health service?

When someone says that the Mona Lisa is the greatest painting in the world, what they actually mean is that they *believe* it is the greatest painting in the world. There is not, nor can there be in most circumstances, an absolute measure of beauty or greatness, any more than there is of quality. The obvious exception is in a competition, where someone can demonstrably be the best in the world or the top person in the class. There are, of course, what might be termed relative absolutes when it comes to quality. The degree of workmanship that goes into a product; the quality of the materials used – a solid beech work surface as opposed to veneer on chipboard; the reliability of a product – though this cannot usually be tested until after purchase; the efficiency of a service. All these are observable and not just to the expert eye.

Can the seller of a product or service truly tell the customer that it is a quality product or service or is it up to the customer to decide? In reality, it does not matter what the seller thinks as he or she is dependent on a purchaser deciding that the product or service is of a quality that meets their needs. But quality, while not an absolute, is not an abstract concept either; it is bound up with price and, even more importantly, with value for money. If you buy a shirt for £3.99, you know you are probably not getting something that is brilliantly made and of the highest quality material which will last for years. But it may suit your purpose. If it falls apart after 6 months, you are not surprised. You may still feel you have derived value for money from it. In other words, the purchaser or customer confers value on a product or service, not the producer or seller. Nor is value an innate attribute within a product or service.

Within the private sector, price is an integral part of the customer's notion of quality, as it is a key factor in the purchase decision. In the NHS, price is not an issue for the customer, who will think an operation is essential whether it costs £1500 or £150 000. Within the service sector, value for money is the key concept and the one underpinning effective communications.

Value for money

In health care, price is an unknown quantity for the patient or client unless they are in the independent sector. In the NHS, patients would not expect a cut-price operation or a cheap consultation – two hips for the price of one, say. They do expect 100% effectiveness in the sense that they are ill and they expect health professionals to get them better. Value for money, on the other hand, is a very clear concept in the NHS. It is, however, a complex and very personal concept. For example, someone who has to wait half an hour for an appointment with a GP may be content to do so if:

- they have brought an enjoyable book to read
- the waiting area is quiet and comfortable
- the GP listens to them, gives them adequate time, is caring and provides an acceptable diagnosis and a cure.

Conversely, they may not be content if:

- the waiting area is noisy and untidy
- they have nothing to do while they wait
- the GP is uncaring, brusque and dismissive.

Any one of these negative aspects could persuade the patient that the service offers poor value. Put simply, the same person who is prepared to queue on the pavement for 2 days in order to get a bargain in the sales may be irritable if they are in a queue for more than 3 minutes at a supermarket checkout. Value for money and quality are inextricably linked in the customer's mind. What then in NHS terms might the customer construe as good or bad quality?

Chapman & Cowdell (1998) equate price with value for money and identify the following as non-monetary factors which are seen as costs by the customer:

- costs associated with the poor image of the public sector
- waiting times for public sector provision

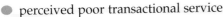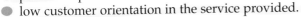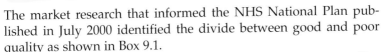

- perceived poor transactional service
- low customer orientation in the service provided.

The market research that informed the NHS National Plan published in July 2000 identified the divide between good and poor quality as shown in Box 9.1.

In summary, quality is what the customer perceives as quality, not the hospital manager or ward sister. Customers define quality in health care in much the same way that they do in the high street, with the exception of price, and their definitions are subjective. If your customers perceive your products as not representing value for money, as a private company you are doomed unless you do something about it. In the health services, increasingly, patients are able to make choices and, with the advent of clinical governance and the National Plan, providers will lose out financially if their quality is seen as poor.

How, then, can a health care provider ensure its customers and potential customers see it as a quality organisation? Being good is not enough; you have to communicate your 'goodness'. On a macro level, that means a stream of 'good news' information that screams quality. This might include:

- a medical breakthrough in your trust
- waiting lists cut or a new initiative to reduce them
- extra/new clinical staff appointed
- new buildings planned/started/completed/opened
- targets met or surpassed
- awards won by individuals or units/the trust
- new clinics services planned/opened
- services expanded
- bureaucracy reduced
- public involvement in the work of the trust/unit.

Each of these pieces of information can be seen as a single brick in the wall of public confidence. No one item will convince patients

Quality communication

Box 9.1

Good quality	Poor quality
Treatment that works	Long wait for a consultation/operation
Practitioners who give them time	Brusque/rude staff
Sympathetic/caring staff	Poor/inadequate hospital food
Quick test results	Long wait for test results
Pleasant environment	Staff not around when needed

that the trust is a quality organisation but, collectively and cumulatively, they will. How this sort of information can be transmitted has been discussed in previous chapters. A critical point is that none of this will be credible unless your staff know what is going on and believe, themselves, that they work for a quality organisation. On a micro level, quality, or lack of it, is perceived through personal contact with the provider.

As already discussed in the context of the £3.99 shirt, people's perceptions of quality are based on their assumptions about the quality they expect. What do health care customers expect? If their expectations are not managed, they may be unrealistic and, therefore, the customers may be disappointed. In health care terms, this is about honesty in relation to prognosis and providing all possible information. Yet how many people waiting to go into hospital for an operation or course of treatment really know what to expect? How many hospitals communicate effectively with their patients beforehand? A home visit to explain the process and procedure, the likely pain, inconvenience or after-effects, the likely recovery time and the longer term prognosis is not only good practice, it also manages the patient's (and their family's) expectations. This is a key element in perceptions of quality. One of the most effective and enduring television advertisements in recent years has been one of the simplest and cheapest: the Ronseal Woodstain advertisement. Its slogan is: 'It does what it says on the tin'. No surprises, no shocks, no unrealistic expectations. Health care should be like that but good communications are required to achieve it.

CUSTOMER SATISFACTION SURVEYS

There can be few people who have never been asked to complete a customer satisfaction survey of one sort or another. What is their purpose, do they always achieve it and can they be counterproductive?

The wider context

Customer satisfaction surveys are a market research tool and market research is big business. Opinion surveys, focus groups and citizens' juries are routinely referred to in newspaper articles without any need to define or explain their purpose. Market research has come out from behind the clipboard into the public arena. Organisations use market research for four main reasons.

- To establish the potential market for a new product.
- To test a new product with current and/or potential customers.
- To find out what existing and/or potential customers think of a current product or service.
- To find out what people think about the organisation's image and reputation.

In essence, market research is about finding out about the present and helping to predict the future. It is about eliminating risk – that existing customers will disappear or that new products or services will fail to enthuse customers.

Customer satisfaction

Customer satisfaction surveys are inherently sensible but they can backfire. Probably the most common form to which we are all exposed is the waiter or waitress asking 'Is everything all right?'. While not a survey as such, it is on the face of it an attempt to gauge customer satisfaction. Unfortunately, it is usually obvious that the question is rhetorical and if you say the food or service is awful, they look startled and are not sure what to do. Customer satisfaction surveys should not be like this if you want to avoid antagonising your customers and are genuinely seeking practical feedback.

There are other pitfalls. I recall a very simple transaction with a bank. Three days later, I received in the post a two-page questionnaire asking me to judge the quality of the service. Most of the questions were irrelevant to my transaction, overcomplicated and rather pointless. That survey did nothing to cement or improve customer relations. So when and how should customer satisfaction surveys be used?

There is no point in undertaking a customer satisfaction survey if you are not prepared to accept customers' verdicts on your service and are not prepared to change the way you do business as a result. Customers know a perfunctory survey when they see one and the public relations fallout can be immense.

In health care settings, there are many aspects of service that can be tested and several ways of testing them. Should you seek to test them all at once or, rather, focus on one or two aspects in depth? An all-encompassing survey can give you a good overall picture of how your customers view the organisation and its services but it is unlikely to be of any use if you want more than a superficial analysis. However, such omnibus surveys are valuable starting points and can help to identify weaknesses for further probing, leading to

Quality communication

action. They are more likely to be of use in testing opinion on the hygiene factors of care rather than the actual treatment. For example, they could be used to test a range of aspects of care provided, such as:

- the appointments booking system
- receptionist service
- waiting area
- patient information
- the episode of care itself
- follow-up information
- navigation around the hospital site
- coordination between different departments.

At the UKCC, we use omnibus surveys every other year to test the views of a 30 000 sample of the register. On the basis of the results, we subsequently focus on anything that requires follow-up work. The 2000 survey highlighted an issue about our quarterly magazine, *Register*, which, while scoring highly for usefulness and relevance, was less positive about readability. Further work was initiated to establish what this meant (see Application 9.1 for more detail).

A more focused customer satisfaction survey might, for example, concentrate solely on the appointments and reception aspects, i.e. before any care takes place. Questioning in depth allows you to go beyond the yes/no answers and the instant judgements in order to explore qualitatively what your patients really think. General feelings of dissatisfaction may not be enough. Having established that all is not well with these aspects of the service via an omnibus survey, an in-depth survey might cover the following questions.

- Did you book your appointment by telephone/post/in person?
- Were you offered a choice of times?
- Were you offered a choice of days/dates?
- Were you told that evening/weekend appointments are available?
- Were you asked if you required help in getting to . . . ?
- Was the receptionist helpful/friendly/polite?
- Did you receive a letter confirming your appointment?
- Did you receive a reminder letter prior to the appointment?
- Were you told precisely where to attend and given a map?
- How long did you have to wait when you arrived for the appointment?

The elements of communication

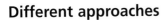

Different approaches

There are different ways of undertaking these surveys. The most common are postal questionnaires, telephone questionnaires and evaluation sheets to be completed on the spot. Each method has its pros and cons.

Method	Advantages	Disadvantages
Postal survey	Time to reflect on answers Easy to analyse if questions are quantitative Large-scale survey possible A good covering letter is a public relations bonus	Expensive on printing and postage Lower response rates
Telephone survey	High response rate Can ask probing questions Personal interaction is good PR if done properly No postal/printing costs	People can be caught out People resent intrusion Cannot do large-scale survey
Evaluation form	Instant answers may provide honest 'gut' reactions No postal costs	People are in a rush to get out Superficial answers People are too close to the episode of care to think properly

There is one other method which, while less structured and quantitative, has the merits of being quick, cheap, simple, non-threatening and good PR. That is just to ask a random selection of patients how they feel about what happened as they are about to leave the clinic. No clipboards and nothing written down, just a friendly chat on their way out.

Whatever method you use, it is essential to provide feedback to participants in any structured survey. This would normally be via a letter, which would remind them that they took part in a survey, thank them for their valuable contribution and feedback, summarise the key findings and, most important of all, **tell them what will happen as a result of the survey**. This latter might be a new appointments system, simpler patient information, a new seating arrangement in the waiting room, etc.

Customer satisfaction surveys are valuable tools in assessing what key people think of the service you provide. You may think your clinic is brilliant but your view is unimportant. It is what your patients think that matters and you need to find this out on a regular basis and not just when something has gone wrong.

NATIONAL INITIATIVES

Hand in hand with the advent of a more patient-centred approach to health care delivery has come a particular emphasis on quality and this can clearly be seen in the national initiatives launched by the Department of Health from the late 1990s onwards. None of these is about communications per se but good communications are critical to all of them in different ways.

The annual reports of the NHS Ombudsman (Health Service Ombudsman 2001) regularly feature complaints by patients and their families which centre on poor communications. People appear to be less concerned about an episode of care going wrong than with the poor communications that may follow. At the same time, it is apparent that there is a great deal of excellent clinical and administrative practice within the NHS in individual clinics and trusts but this is not communicated to other providers. The new national initiatives are largely designed to remedy these shortcomings. The National Institute for Clinical Excellence and the Commission for Health Improvement are chiefly about good clinical practice. The two initiatives to be discussed in greater depth deal with organisational aspects of health care delivery and customer orientation.

Clinical governance

The concept of clinical governance was formally and statutorily introduced into the NHS in 1998. For the first time, clear accountabilities were established in statute for, for example, the chief executives of trusts, while existing processes for quality assurance and audit were brought together in one framework. That framework includes functions and values such as professional regulation, good communication, patient focus and a commitment to quality. Good communications with patients and between colleagues are an ineluctable part of clinical governance.

NHS National Plan

Before the dust had settled on the introduction of clinical governance, and while practitioners and managers were still grappling with its implications, the government published its national plan for the NHS in July 2000. This strategy document embodies customer orientation. The first chapter is entitled 'Our vision: a health service designed around the patient'. Throughout the plan are references to the need for better communication. That means better communication between:

- the different professions
- different teams
- patients and administrators
- patients and doctors
- health and social services.

While new structures will provide the framework for these better communications, it will be the day-to-day communications that ensure their delivery. The prerequisites for this will include:

- better and more user-friendly trust intranets for staff
- less bureaucratic and more useful patient-focused communication
- communication that breaks down barriers between professions and teams
- greater use of customer satisfaction surveys and other market research.

National initiatives of any kind and by any government may be the foundations for better quality communications but the bricks and mortar will be the day-to-day communications efforts that will influence patient perceptions of the health care they receive. Organisations cannot change from being systems oriented to customer oriented overnight but patients will recognise and appreciate even the smallest indications that their needs are being put first.

CONCLUSION

Being treated as a customer does not mean that patients are no longer patients; they are both. Building your organisation and its communications strategy around your customers – a customer orientation – means you are more likely to meet their needs. That will lead to greater customer satisfaction and fewer complaints. Customer satisfaction can and should be measured on a regular

Quality communication

basis but only if you are prepared to change the way you do business as a result of what customers say.

Customers recognise good and bad quality when they see it, whether they are purchasing a tangible product or receiving a service. A substantial element within that judgement is the notion of value for money, which is subjective and based largely on their personal experience of your service provision. Overall judgements about the quality of an organisation, hospital or clinic can and should be influenced over time through the effective and positive communication of success, improvement and achievement.

Practice checklist

- All organisations have customers and stakeholders, not just those in the commercial world. Your patients and clients are your customers. Each contact with them influences their perceptions of the organisation. The speed, efficiency and courtesy with which that contact is made – the hygiene factors – are key factors in determining customer satisfaction.
- NHS trusts generally epitomise systems-oriented organisations. Putting your customers at the heart of your practice may require a substantial cultural shift in attitude on the part of all trust staff.
- Customer satisfaction surveys are useful tools in gauging what your customers think of your service. They can be qualitative or quantitative, small scale or comprehensive. By finding out what customers think, you will be able to deliver an appropriate service in a customer-oriented way.
- Health care organisations should be no less cognisant of how their customers judge the services they provide than any commercial company. The critical issue is the value-for-money rating that customers ascribe to your service.

Discussion questions

- Do you see your patients as your customers? How is that manifested on a daily basis?
- What is needed to transform your organisation/practice from systems orientation to customer orientation? What can you contribute to that transformation?
- Are there differences between how you perceive your organisation/practice and how your customers see it?
- How does your experience as a health care provider compare with your experience as a patient?

The elements of communication

References

Chapman D, Cowdell T 1998 New public sector marketing. Financial Times/ Pitman Publishing, London

Department of Health 2000 The NHS Plan: a plan for investment, a plan for reform. Stationery Office, London

Health Service Ombudsman 2001 Investigations completed December 2000– March 2001. Stationery Office, London

Mitroff II 1983 Stakeholders of the organisational mind. Jossey-Bass, San Francisco, California

Morgan C, Murgatroyd S 1994 Total quality management in the public sector. Open University Press, Buckingham

Further reading

Chapman D, Cowdell T 1998 New public sector marketing. Financial Times/ Pitman Publishing, London

Morgan C, Murgatroyd S 1994 Total quality management in the public sector. Open University Press, Buckingham

Silver R 1985 Health service public relations: a guide to good practice. King's Fund Publishing, London

Walker H, Richardson J 1986 Marketing. Pan, London, Sydney

Quality communication

Application 9:1

Stuart Skyte

Customer satisfaction surveys

INTRODUCTION

This chapter examines three examples of customer satisfaction survey: one is an omnibus survey, testing customers' awareness, understanding, knowledge and perceptions of the organisation. Another tested an organisation's core communications services, while the third examined one particular aspect of an organisation's communications to its key customers. The chapter looks at how each survey was undertaken, the main findings and the actions taken as a result.

AN OMNIBUS SURVEY

The UKCC undertook an omnibus survey in 1996/97 to establish the perceptions and awareness of a key 'customer'. As the regulatory body for the three professions, the UKCC sees practitioners as key customers and stakeholders, yet it had not until then undertaken such a large-scale piece of market research.

Using an out-house market research company, a three-stage approach was adopted: a telephone survey, followed by a 30 000 postal survey, followed in turn by another telephone survey. Why three separate surveys? Before undertaking a written questionnaire, you have to be certain that the questions asked will elicit the answers you want in that they will be useful, measureable and actionable. That means the questions should be almost exclusively quantitative. For example, to establish quantitatively how practitioners saw the UKCC, a small number were asked by telephone to provide three words describing the organisation. These were then bracketed together to establish eight key words for the written questionnaire. These included 'efficient, remote, bureaucratic and accessible'. Once all the questionnaires had been analysed, a further telephone survey was used to probe some of the answers. For example, it was established that people wanted more information about the UKCC, but what?

In summary form, the key stages for an omnibus survey could be as follows.

1. Draft written questionnaire.
2. Write to a small number to say you are telephoning them and why.
3. Use the telephone survey to firm up the written questions.
4. Send out the questionnaire with a detailed covering letter, personally addressed, explaining why/how they have been selected, the purpose of the survey and the confidentiality, and promising a summary of the results. Include a reply-paid envelope.
5. Follow up any grey areas with a telephone survey.
6. Write to thank everyone who took part and enclose a summary of the findings.

The UKCC's omnibus survey highlighted the fact that, while practitioners saw it as an efficient and valuable organisation, they also saw it as remote. To counter that, the organisation trebled the number of roadshows around the UK, doubled the frequency of its news magazine, held more open days and produced new publicity leaflets about its work. A follow-up survey in 1999/2000 showed that the change had paid off in terms of perceptions. There was a marked reduction in the numbers seeing the UKCC as remote.

Testing core communications services

An organisation wanted to establish what a key group of customers with whom it had regular contact – by post, telephone and automated systems – felt about those systems. Were they seen as efficient, customer-friendly systems and were there areas that could be improved? At the same time, the survey was used to refresh customer orientation within the organisation, which had seen a number of new staff recruited in the previous year.

A brief questionnaire was sent out to a customer sample. This included questions on the telephone system, the website, the response to written requests for information, satisfaction with an advice line and so on. A response rate of over 60% was considered high and a reflection of the goodwill existing between the organisation and this group of customers. The questionnaire was used both to elicit information and promote new services.

Customer satisfaction surveys

Surveys can be used to promote aspects of an organisation's services or products. If you ask a question to establish whether customers know that you provide a particular service, if they didn't before, they do now!

As a result of the survey, new ways of ordering goods were considered, the backlog of orders was cleared, some extant publications were reissued, a new complaints system was considered, a new series of meetings with key customers was established and the internal standards of business, covering, for example, turnround times for correspondence, were revised.

A specific aspect of communications tested

A public body in the health care field had used a particular form of formal communication with a key set of customers for many years. It wanted to test whether the information sent out was considered useful and relevant, whether the tone and style were appropriate and what customers did with the information. A short questionnaire was sent to 10% of these customers.

The results were very satisfactory in that 92% said the information was useful, 85% said the style and tone were about right and 81% said there was the right amount of detail. More than 80% of recipients passed the information to others. Two-thirds were not yet ready to receive information via email.

While no immediate action was necessary, it is likely that the organisation will have followed up at regular intervals to test the use of email communication with this group of customers.

In addition to promoting specific products or services, such surveys can have a significant public relations value. The very fact that you are seeking your customers' opinions and are committed to responding to them is a major plus point.

You might like to consider the following questions.

- What sort of response rate might be considered reasonable in a customer satisfaction survey?
- What factors might influence the response rate (either way)?
- When should you use a large-scale survey and when would a small one suffice?
- How do you ensure that staff are comfortable with a survey that could be construed as testing their efficiency?

Action plans

Select one aspect of the services you provide and devise a pilot customer satisfaction survey. Test it out on a small number of colleagues and a few customers. Draw up an action plan when you have analysed the results and discuss this with colleagues.

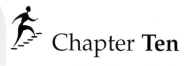 Chapter **Ten**

Information technology and systems in communication

Mike Tatlow

The elements of communication

- **Background**
- **Communication, organisations and the NHS**
- **The information technology network**

- **Telephone**
- **Facsimile (fax)**
- **Email and associated technologies**

O V E R V I E W

This chapter covers the technical aspects of communication and differs from the other chapters in that it does not focus on individuals and how they communicate. This said, it is important to note that technical devices to speed up or assist communication are becoming more and more prevalent in our working and personal lives. In spite of this and the amazement we express at being able to communicate almost instantaneously, by email for example, this is often tempered by the ease with which an email can cause offence or simply be misinterpreted. Mike Tatlow considers these issues by reminding us that even though technology serves up wonder after wonder the key to effective use lies in getting the human element right.

A range of technical information is also offered in relation to data protection and the way in which information technology systems work and affect our lives. Readers will be able to pick and choose what level of detail they require but this comprehensive chapter covers a vast array of information on behalf of the clinical professional.

INTRODUCTION

This chapter aims to review the mechanics behind the communication methods employed in business and, more importantly, the etiquette and protocols for the effective and efficient use of new and emerging technologies in the health care arena. Being able to use the available technologies effectively and possessing an awareness of the appropriateness of each will serve the health care practitioner well in communicating information and knowledge to others.

BACKGROUND

Communication in any organisation is critical to its success and well-being. For the organisation to fully exploit the potential of communication and therefore achieve its purpose it must fully understand the various types of mechanisms available and how they figure in the wider overview of data and information exchange. The how and why of the exchange of information between individuals and groups is much dependent on the physical location of the users.

To help in an understanding of such communication mechanisms it is perhaps useful to explore a chronology of business communication.

Information and its uses have always constituted a measure of power of an organisation or country. The Church of the Middle Ages controlled the production of written media and therefore wielded a significant amount of power, along with the monarchy. In the Middle Ages, Guttenberg and the printing press provided a mechanism for disseminating knowledge and information more widely, thus heralding the beginning of the modern information age. It could be said that Guttenberg was the first informaticist.

From the print medium through voice to data communication, the use of transmission technologies has aided in the dispersal of knowledge and information.

The commercial world has traditionally embraced information and communication technologies (ICT) earlier and more effectively than the health care and education sectors. This can be seen as primarily driven by financial consideration and pressures. It has long been stated that 'information is power'. In the late 1990s, central government recognised the potential inequality resulting from not being able to access the Internet. John Prescott, the Deputy Prime Minister at the time, announced a plan to provide second user personal computers to families in the low-income

Information technology and systems in communication

bracket in an attempt to give everyone an opportunity to access the Internet.

Industry has certainly embraced and proven the concept of information power, especially in the field of ICT. The Microsoft Corporation is one example of how providing the tools for successful exchange of data and information has enabled a commercial organisation to grow and become as, if not more, powerful than individual countries.

Commerce relies heavily on the successful transfer of information between individuals and groups within the organisation and with other organisations and institutions.

COMMUNICATION, ORGANISATIONS AND THE NHS

To achieve a well-structured method of communication within an organisation, acknowledgement should be made of how, why and what information the members of the organisation pass between each other and to the outside world.

In the health care arena there are differing levels and needs for information transfer. The simplest dataset is plain text and the most demanding is the storage, transmission and displaying of medical images in specialisms such as radiography. The highest demands for both the network and processing power should be viewed as the minimum specification needed for the network.

The current concept for the infrastructure for linking of sites within the National Health Service and the methods to be used are based on the White Paper *Information for health* (1998). This paper identifies methods and structures for the exchange of information between organisations within the NHS and includes such features as:

- network infrastructure – a stand-alone isolated national network
- communication protocols for data, voice and electronic messaging
- NHSWeb – a NHS Internet protocol-based national secure intranet supported by the stand-alone network
- 'open' access to data
- NHS Information Authority – an organisation evolved from the NHSIM&T strategy
- NICE – National Institute for Clinical Excellence
- NeLH – National Electronic Library for Health

The elements of communication

- authentication – weak and strong, trusted third parties
- code of connection.

These features are slowly taking shape. NICE has already begun to impact on the realm of evidence-based practice and this, allied to the development of the National Electronic Library for Health, has provided the resources for health care practitioners to enhance reflective practice. This has been essential with the development of clinical governance. The network infrastructure is becoming a reality for many trusts and this is having a positive impact on data exchange between departments within hospitals and with organisations such as primary care teams outside the hospital structure.

Information and legislation

When information is passed between individuals in a health organisation, it becomes subject to a series of government Acts. The main statutes affecting health information and data are derivatives of the Data Protection Act – Protection and Use of Patient Information 1998 which is an enhancement of the original Data Protection Act of 1984.

There are primarily four statutes that give a subject access to information about them held by the NHS; the statutes provide a framework for the appropriate handling of such data.

- The *Data Protection Act 1984* which, with some exemptions, entitles individuals to a copy of computerised information held about them. Repealed in 1998.
- The *Access to Personal Files Act 1987*, which concerns personal information held by local authority social services and may therefore be relevant in cases of joint care.
- The *Access to Medical Reports Act 1988*, in respect of reports for employers and insurance companies.
- The *Access to Health Records Act 1990*, in respect of an individual's access to health records.

The Data Protection Act 1998 – Protection and Use of Patient Information seeks to combine all the previous pieces of legislation and supersedes the Data Protection Act 1984.

The Data Protection Act 1984

The original Data Protection Act established a number of principles to which any organisation recording and retaining electronic information about patients and individuals had to adhere. This was the first attempt by government to establish a degree of protection for the individual. Unfortunately it did not fully address the needs of systems even then and a series of further pieces of legislation followed that directly affected the way information about an individual was dealt with.

Access to Health Records Act 1990

This Act aimed to address the more specific needs of the health care sector. It was expected to fill some of the gaps which were evident within the earlier 1984 Act but it still had significant failings. One of these was that the Act only had control over electronic records and the traditional written records fell outside the Act's jurisdiction.

The Data Protection Act 1998 – Protection and Use of Patient Information

This Act, which came into effect on 1 March 2000, possesses many similarities to the original Act but there are significant changes.

- The Act now covers certain types of manual records (including all health records) as well as electronic records.
- There are transitional arrangements concerning manual records between now and 2007; the definition of 'processing' is wider than that in the 1984 Act and includes the concept of 'obtaining'.
- Storing and disclosing data. Most actions involving data, including storage, will be included within this definition. Although both the 1984 and 1998 Act include eight Data Protection Principles the nature of the principles differs radically. One such change is the inclusion of handwritten medical records under the Act rather than the exclusion of such records, therefore permitting access to them by patients.
- Differences between the two Acts. The Access to Health Records Act 1990 permitted access to manual health records made after the Act came into force (1 November 1991). The Data Protection Act 1998 permits access to all manual health records.
- Access to manual records is subject to specified exceptions. This includes changes to the requirements for notification of processing to the Data Protection Commissioner (formerly the Data Protection Registrar).

The Act also encompasses new data protection principles. All processing of data to which the Act applies must comply with eight principles. The first principle is particularly important as it empha-

The elements of communication

sises that processing must be fair and lawful in the context of the common law and other UK legislation. Generally it will be complied with if the common law of confidentiality and any other applicable statutory restrictions on the use of information have been met. These include the following.

- The data subject was not misled or deceived into giving the data.
- The data subject is given basic information about who will process the data and for what purpose.
- In the case of health data, one of the conditions in both Schedules 2 and 3 to the Act is satisfied. Schedule 2 conditions apply to the processing of all personal data. More stringent protection is provided for sensitive data, which include data about racial or ethnic origin, physical or mental health or condition and sexual life. Processing of such data must meet one of the conditions of not only Schedule 2 but also Schedule 3. One of those conditions is that the processing is necessary for 'medical purposes', which is not defined exhaustively but includes preventative medicine, medical diagnosis, medical research, provision of care and treatment and the management of health care services.
- 'Processing' of the data is widely defined and covers all manner of use including obtaining, recording, holding, altering, retrieving, destroying or disclosing data.
- Data processing for legitimate NHS purposes is likely to satisfy one or more of the conditions set out in Schedules 2 and 3; in particular, the conditions set out at Schedule 2(6) and at Schedule 3(8) appear relevant. In addition, the Data Protection (Processing of Sensitive Personal Data) Order 2000 provides further conditions under which it will be lawful to process sensitive personal data. Lawful processing under the 1998 Act requires compliance with the common-law duty of confidentiality where patient data are concerned. Guidance on this can be found in HSG (96) 18, The Protection and Use of Patient Information.
- Data subjects should be informed of the identity of the data controller (this will usually be the NHS body), the purposes for which data are to be processed and any other information needed to make the processing fair (see paragraph 2(3) (d) of Part II of Schedule 1). Where the data were not obtained from the data subject himself, there is an exemption from the requirement to provide this information where providing it would involve disproportionate effort or data are obtained or used

pursuant to a non-contractual legal requirement. However, if the ground of disproportionate effort is to be relied on then the provisions of the Data Protection (Conditions under Paragraph 3 of Part II of Schedule 1) Order 2000 must also be met. As required by HSG (96) 18, The Protection and Use of Patient Information, NHS bodies should seek to ensure that patients are informed of the potential use of their data in general terms.

Individuals are entitled to prevent processing:

- for direct marketing purposes; it is Department of Health policy that patient information should not be disclosed for such purposes
- which will, or is likely to, cause the data subject or another person unwarranted and substantial harm or distress. This right can be overridden in certain circumstances, including:
  - where the processing is necessary to meet contractual obligations to which the data subject is a party or to enter a contract at the latter's request
  - where it is necessary to protect the data subject's vital interests
  - where it is necessary for compliance with the data controller's non-contractual legal obligations.

Any data subject who suffers damage due to an unauthorised disclosure is entitled to compensation, although a data controller will have a defence if reasonable care was taken to comply with the Act.

There are a number of codes of practices outlining what information can and cannot be provided to organisations outside the NHS.

THE INFORMATION TECHNOLOGY NETWORK

The physical layers, the cables and hardware, which support the software communication structure traditionally, exist within the physical fabric of the buildings of an organisation. They help form the network that physically connects the various pieces of the organisation together.

Unfortunately, the National Health Service has a large number of old computer systems that have historically answered communication and storage needs for individual departments. However, they have not been able to interact and participate in the exchange of information between other departments and within the wider organisation. Attempts to link the disparate infrastructures have been partially successful, the physical cabling having been linked and shown to communicate. However, the software and 'applications' have proven more difficult. This non-communication has proved an obstacle to the creation of a seamless 'open' communication network within and between NHS trusts.

Historically, telephone and data communication networks have been kept separate from each other which has proved to be a handicap. A computer network traditionally had a copper (cable) based infrastructure. More recently, demands for an integrated infrastructure have lead to combining data and voice communications across a single network – 'multiplexing'. This has enabled a single network to support the communication needs of an organisation.

In the day-to-day business environment, the range of methods available to users to communicate with each other includes:

- face to face – voice
- telephone – voice
- fax – data/documents
- electronic mail – data/documents.

In the business world, with its requirement for speed and accuracy, the ability to make a favourable impression gives one the edge over potential competitors. In health care, the need for speed, accuracy and confidentiality has produced current protocols and infrastructure and has driven the development of legislation. This encompasses voice, text and data.

TELEPHONE

When we converse in face-to-face situations, we rely on non-verbal as well as verbal communication. A person's body language, facial expression and tone of voice all add to the interaction. In a telephone conversation, two of these three components are removed so we need to use other techniques to portray our feelings, ideas and demeanour.

Telephone etiquette

We have all called a company and spoken to someone who was very unhelpful, discourteous or completely ignorant about the organisation's operations. Unfortunately, these situations occur frequently but that does not mean that they are appropriate ways to conduct professional conversations. So how do we give the listener the correct impression?

The caller's first impression of the organisation or individual is established by the greeting. Consequently, it is important that the greeting is polite, positive and professional.

It is advisable that all calls are answered by the second ring and the caller is greeted with the following:

- a goodwill message such as 'good morning' or 'good afternoon'
- the name of the organisation
- your name and designation, if appropriate
- a statement of assistance, such as 'How can I help you?'.

The tone of your voice can be used to build goodwill with the caller; smile as you speak and callers will 'hear' your smile through your friendly tone of voice (it does work!). This will put them at ease, especially if they are calling with a complaint. Never use an annoyed or hostile tone of voice, regardless of how frustrating the call may be.

Having respect for the caller also helps in gaining their confidence and establishing a working rapport so avoid negative behaviours such as:

- interrupting the caller
- expressing hostility in your voice
- using vulgar language
- allowing yourself to be distracted from the call.

During the conversation you should attempt to make the caller your number one priority, thinking about their needs and how their interest can be maintained. This is of particular importance when we consider the interactions between health care professionals and patients.

If there is a need to put a caller 'on hold' while you search for further information or to enquire whether a particular person is available, ask for the caller's permission. Simply ask the caller 'May I put you on hold for a moment?' or 'Can you please hold?'. Some callers may be unable to do so, especially if they are calling long distance. Therefore, offer an alternative such as returning this call when you have the necessary information or available person. If the caller can hold, check back with the caller every 15–20 seconds to show that you have not abandoned them. In certain situations this may not be possible but be aware that the caller may have been 'holding' for some time and apologise for the delay and offer to call them back.

If you need to transfer a caller, be sure you transfer the call and not the caller. In other words, don't make a transfer simply because you do not like the person on the other end. Only after you have determined that you are unable to assist the caller with their needs should you transfer the call. In addition, inform the caller that they are being transferred and inform the recipient of the call as to the situation.

Speaker phones

These have been a boon to telephone communications as they allow the communicator to talk while they move about their office or introduce others into the conversation. Though these features are regarded as a benefit, they also come with a significant number of dangers.

They require a more open approach to the conversation, remembering that the other caller can hear what is being said in the immediate area of the phone.

Conference calls

Conference calls enable the linking up of more than one caller to a conversation. This is normally facilitated by a digital exchange and requires no special telephone equipment but a set procedure needs to be followed which is normally detailed by the telephone service provider.

A conference call allows remote parties to establish a group conversation and have a meeting. It does incur a higher call cost but this is normally outweighed by the cost saving in terms of time and travel for the people to meet face to face.

Mobile phones

These are probably the most controversial piece of technology to be introduced in the last 10 years. They have had significant impact in all areas of society, providing significant freedom to individuals in terms of communication.

They have been subject to research from both ends of the safety spectrum and have been proven to be a danger in the medical environment where the radiation from a mobile phone has been shown to affect implanted pacemakers (Trigano et al 1999).

The technology of the wireless phone is relatively new but because of rapid changes in the industry, what we call it may need to be updated fairly often. Cellular phone, digital phone, car phone, wireless phone or mobile phone . . . the biggest complaint is

Information technology and systems in communication

233

not what we call it. How and when the mobile phone is used is a significant source of contention and upset.

Some states in the USA are planning to legislate as to how and where mobile phones are used. (As of 1 January 2000, California has required hands-free operation when driving a car.) How can we avoid the finger wagging being directed at us? A little consideration is the answer.

There are places and times when we should not use our wireless communication mechanisms (phone or pager):

- funeral or wedding service
- other religious service
- movie
- theatre performance
- business meeting
- meal with clients
- meal with friends (restaurant or private home).

Ideally your telephone (and pager) ringer should be turned off and have the storage capability to save any messages for later retrieval.

It is sometimes necessary to make (or take) an important call for business reasons because the recipient is only available at that specified time. In recent times the making of a call has become an irritant and we should avoid offending people in close proximity. There are four steps to being considerate in this situation.

- First, explain and apologise in advance to colleagues that you are expecting to take or make the call at a particular time and that it is unavoidable.
- Second, excuse yourself during the call to a quiet outdoor place or private room or near the public telephones.
- Third, keep it brief and your voice low.
- Return to your party with a sincere apology.

Driving and making mobile phone calls is both against the law and potentially dangerous. Many police forces take a dim view of those using the telephone whilst behind the steering wheel of a car.

If you must use a mobile phone whilst driving there are two solutions.

- The least expensive accessory for hands-free use is the external cord variety that has a tiny earpiece and microphone to clip to your collar. Calls are surprisingly clear at both ends of the system but remember to lower the radio and consider other car passengers who can be heard by your caller via the floating microphone.

- The more expensive option for hands-free use is having the speaker, microphone and car phone holder professionally mounted in your car by the speciality store or service garage.

Remember, hands-free capability does not mean you have a hand free to write down the information someone gives you over the phone, in your day planner on the passenger seat, while you are driving. If the caller wishes to give you a message, suggest they leave the information on your office/home answering machine and you can pick it up when you are not driving.

Answerphones

Answerphones and voicemail are methods of recording messages from callers. In function they possess the same attributes but they differ in how they are accessed by the user.

Answerphones traditionally have been placed next to or formed part of the desk telephone. They possess an external speaker so the user is able to hear what the incoming caller is saying, making call screening possible. Voicemail, however, is integral to the telephone system itself. The user diverts the incoming call to a central answering service where the calls are logged and messages recorded. The user accesses the saved messages via a single number or button. Some systems indicate on the user's telephone that there is a call waiting to be dealt with but this is not true of all systems.

Many voicemail systems and some modern answerphones come with a standard system greeting. This should be viewed as an emergency option and all users should be encouraged to create a personalised greeting, which should contain at least the following information:

- organisation name
- user name and title
- an alternative contact name and extension – make sure this is normally a person, **not** another answerphone or voicemail
- the date when the message was set.

The message should also reflect vacation and sickness days, training or travel, dates of departure and return. In the case of unexpected absence, the current message should suffice.

Updating of the outgoing message should be performed as circumstances change and recorded messages should be checked at least three times each day.

Information technology and systems in communication

FACSIMILE (FAX)

The fax or, more correctly, facsimile machine makes use of three types of computer peripheral: the scanner, the modem and the printer. In recent times it has, to a certain extent, been superseded by email which allows documents in both their raw form (such as a word processor document) and in protected form (such as Adobe Acrobat format) to be transferred between users quickly and cheaply.

Fax has become a well-used and accepted mechanism for transferring documents between remote sites. Like the telephone, it should be used within a protocol.

● Send the fax when promised. Your credibility suffers if your fax is not received on time. It can also act as a source of irritation to the intended recipient.

● Always include a cover sheet. For convenience and clarity, the cover should state the recipient's name, telephone number, fax number and department. It should also include your name, phone number, fax number and indicate the number of pages being sent. This information will enable you to be contacted should the intended fax number be incorrectly dialled.

● Give your fax the same professional appearance as your other correspondence. Just because it is a fax does not mean that it should be any less professional. Many institutions have templates for fax cover sheets.

● Include a confidentiality disclaimer: *The contents of this facsimile are confidential. It may not be disclosed to, or used by, anyone other than the addressee. If you receive this facsimile in error, please destroy its contents and advise the sender immediately.*

● Notify the recipient by telephone that a fax has been sent. In many large companies a fax can easily become lost in the system. It could be hours or days before the fax gets to the intended recipient which can be a problem when sending time-sensitive or confidential documents.

● Beware of sending more than three or four pages by fax. Unless you have been requested to do so, sending a lengthy document can tie up a fax line unnecessarily. This is particularly important when the phone and fax line are the same. Notify the recipient that you are sending a lengthy fax and ask permission. This provides an opportunity for the recipient to suggest an alternative number or to ask for the document to be sent at a particular time.

The elements of communication

EMAIL AND ASSOCIATED TECHNOLOGIES

Introduction

Recent years have seen an increase in the use and acceptability of electronic data communications, from the facsimile machine to the more pervasive email. Many authors (Sherwood 2000) regard email as a significant advance in personal and business communication. Sherwood (2000) views email as 'cheaper and faster than a letter, less intrusive than a telephone call and less hassle than a fax'. The use of email overcomes the barriers of distance and time and can act as an equaliser in the business field.

Just as we can regard the telephone conversation as being one-third of a face-to-face communication, the email message is significantly less. Communication between humans is approximately 90% body language, 8% tone of voice and 2% what you say. With email, you remove the first 98%.

Be aware of this when you write emails. Be very obvious with your meanings, since subtleties will be lost or completely misunderstood. Remember this, too, when reading others' emails. Their grasp of the language or their haste in composing the email may have given it a 'virtual tone' that may seem derogatory or aggressive. Reread it and see if you are simply misinterpreting the words.

At times, it can be very difficult to determine a sender's demeanour from the text of their email. Always remember that text is unable to impart tone and you, the sender, need to do something in your message to identify your attitude. This is often done with smiles, such as :) or :-).

Composing a message

When composing a message, consideration should be given to typing errors as they can make messages virtually unreadable. Also, be aware of spelling and grammar. We all need to check the spelling and grammar of our messages, first by simply running a spellchecker, then by quickly reviewing the message again for punctuation and grammar. Little typos aren't too worrying but massive typos and run-on sentences tend to be less thoroughly read and go to the bottom of a folder.

Thought needs to be given to how a reader will view the message. A large body of text with no punctuation or application of paragraph style will encourage the reader to skip tracts of text and therefore potentially miss crucial information.

Information technology and systems in communication

237

The email process is the basis of other associated mechanisms: discussion groups, computer-mediated conferences (CMCs), mail lists (and groups) and newsgroups. All of these mechanisms rely on textual input from users to be successful and functional. They are based on the creation of data.

The speed of the delivery can be regarded as almost instantaneous which leads to a feeling that one must respond with similar rapidity. This feeling must be overcome and controlled. Simply responding to a message or sending a message without really thinking about what has been written invites trouble. The world of email is littered with stories of employees sending indiscriminate messages to a mailing list, the recipients of which are senior members of their management team. This leads to embarrassing situations and revelations!

Due to the immediacy of email, people are often quick to write replies or original emails. This is all right when you have something quick to say, like 'Happy Birthday', but when you are upset or furious, the ease of pressing the SEND button can get you into a lot of trouble. If you are upset and want to compose an email, you can write it as hastily as you wish. But don't click the SEND button when you are finished. Instead, let the email sit for an hour or so before sending it. When you return, review the email and make the changes you feel are appropriate, now that you have more composure.

Avoid spraying messages around. If you want to mail a large number of people (for instance, on a mailing list) don't paste all the names into the 'CC' field of your email program. If you do that, all the people you are writing to will be able to see the email addresses of all the other people. This can be very annoying, as people usually do not like to disclose their email address in public. Always use 'BCC' (blind carbon copy) instead. That way, each person will only see his or her own email address on your message.

Many companies require the inclusion of a disclaimer statement at the end of email messages. A suggested form of the message is given below.

> This email is confidential. It may not be disclosed to, or used by, anyone other than the addressee. If you receive this message in error, please advise the sender immediately.

Emails should be written with consideration and some reflection. They are regarded as having the same legal standing as a printed document and are therefore subject to the same areas of litigation.

Treat email confidentially. If somebody sends you information or ideas by email, you should not take it as a licence to post that

The elements of communication

information in a public forum (discussion group, USENET newsgroup, chat site, etc.). Email is one to one for a reason: it is often used for personal communication. Unless you are explicitly told otherwise, always assume that any email you receive has a big 'PRIVATE' sticker on it . . . and don't spread it around.

When replying to a person's email do not overquote; if you are quoting somebody's message in your reply, try to quote only the relevant portions of the message and not the whole thing.

Emails are regarded as transient communications and if they are required as a record they should be printed out and stored in the 'normal' manner.

Do not use ALL UPPER CASE LETTERS

On the Net, the use of all upper case is seen as SHOUTING. Typographers have long known that proper capitalisation makes text easier to read so don't be rude, use the proper case.

Use an appropriate subject line

While it might be nearly impossible to handle 200 telephone calls a day and get anything else accomplished, many people get hundreds of email messages a day. To improve the odds of your message being handled correctly (or even read at all) be sure to use a short and appropriate subject line such as 'Examination Results' or 'Conference Schedule'. If you don't use a subject line or use an inappropriate one, you run the risk of your mail being overlooked.

Modern email programs allow authors to use plain text or HTML. Newer email client packages, including Microsoft Outlook and Netscape Communicator, have the capability to send and receive email in HTML form; that is to say, as a web page. Messages can contain all elements of a web page, including graphics, forms, interactive content, etc. If you send a message in HTML format and the recipient is unable to view HTML mail with their program, your message will look something like this:

```
<HTML>
<HEAD>
<TITLE>HTML Mail! WooWoo!</TITLE>
</HEAD>
<BODY BGCOLOR= "#FFFFFF">
<H1>Patrick-<BR>
<BR>
```

Information technology and systems in communication

```
<HR ALIGN=CENTER SIZE="3" WIDTH="95%"></H1>Look at
this! It's a <FONT COLOR="#FF0000">message</FONT> in
<FONT COLOR="#008080">HTML</FONT>! Pretty neat, eh? It
can have images, <I><U>styled text</U></I>, and much,
much more. I hope you like it!<BR>
<HR ALIGN=CENTER SIZE="3" WIDTH="95%"><BR>
See ya,<BR>
<H2><I><U><BR>
Jeff</U></I></H2>
</BODY>
</HTML>
```

Use a signature, but keep it under six lines

In order to ease the strain of typing your name at the bottom of every email message, you can tell your email software to sign all your messages with a standard signature that is stored in a separate file.

Anything over six lines and the reader will start losing interest. Keep it succinct. Some commentators regard the six-line limit as generous. Newsgroups and mailing lists that accept subscribers' posts often have strict rules about the length of signature files – many say four lines is the maximum allowed.

Viruses and other dangers

In accessing an email system, you open your PC to attack from malicious messages. These range from viruses that directly attack a computer system and are normally contained in an innocent-looking message or attachment to a 'macro' virus which exploits the facility offered by the Microsoft family of products to program functions into documents. These pose a greater threat than conventional viruses as they possess the potential to attack both Windows and Apple Macintosh-based systems. This is a new phenomenon for Apple users as hither to they have had a safe existence compared with Windows users.

How to protect your personal computer

Users can take steps to protect the integrity of the files and machines. Some basic precautions are listed below.

- Do not pass floppy disks between machines.
- Does the sender normally send you attachments?
- Does the sender normally send you files of this type?

- Give the sender a call if you have any doubts.
- Save any suspect attachments in a secure area.
- Maintain up-to-date antivirus software.
- Keep an eye on the headlines and the websites of antivirus vendors, such as*:

www.networkassociates.com
www.symantec.com/avcenter
www.cai.com/virusinfo
www.kasperkylabs.com
www.viruslist.com

Searching the Internet

The invention of World Wide Web (3W) technologies by Tim Berners-Lee in the late 1980s has had the biggest impact on the arena of business communications. Originally developed as a mechanism for the different partners of the European Atomic Energy Commission to communicate and share documents and information, it has become the basis for major commercial concerns. It has provided an 'open' architecture, which allows communication of data and information across the globe in a matter of seconds.

This easy access to the knowledge held on the 3W has brought with it its own peculiar type of problems. Anyone who has basic computing skills and access to the Internet can establish a professional-looking site. These can sometimes be mistaken for the bona fide sites of organisations and professional bodies. There is no mechanism for the validation of site content.

Searching for what you want

When users begin to search the Internet, they visit one of the many 'search engines' present on the 3W. They enter in the topic or term they are searching for and press the SEARCH button. What happens next is almost too predictable! The search engine presents the searcher with '650 000' hits but no indication of what each site holds or the relevance to the search topic.

This weakness has given rise to several Internet portals which review the content of Internet sites. One such site is BioMedNet

---

* It must be noted that the site addresses listed in this chapter were correct at the time of going to press but due to the dynamic nature of the World Wide Web, they may change.

(http://www.bmn.com) which provides access to peer-reviewed Internet sites and will search from its own database for other suitable sites. The benefit to researchers is that they can be confident that the information held on the Internet site is from a bona fide source.

One main source of information for the health researcher regarding central government and health policy is the Department of Health 3W site (see Resources).

Time is the most valuable commodity a researcher has and the development of a successful strategy for searching can significantly reduce the time spent accessing the Internet.

Background knowledge

To be successful in searching for information on the Internet, we need to have an idea of what is and what isn't part of the topic area. Some key points are:

- understand the potential and limitations of the medium
- find something relevant using a broad search
- learn the deep or advanced search techniques
- collect specialist resources in your area
- maintain current awareness – and an awareness strategy
- share your knowledge – and share others'.

Searching techniques

There are several strategies one can employ to speed and refine the search.

- Boolean search methods.
- Know your topic – a familiarity with the content.
- Use on-line sources for further ideas – use the material to feed more ideas into your search.
- Use specialist indexes – these can presearch the material. Searching a medical site for medical information will be quicker than a general search.

Search engines, meta search engines, subject gateways and directories

There are primarily four types of databases held on the 3W.

- *Search engines* – search the Internet dynamically from their own data. Normally a single site.
- *Meta search engines* – search the search engines; one site can search all the different search engines.
- *Subject gateway* – normally a subject database sorted by content.

Can be quicker than a search engine. Gives access to other subject-specific material.

● *Directories* – lists of Internet sites; normally do not show content.

Preparing a search

When we begin to search it is useful to clarify in our minds exactly what we are looking for. Some suggested steps are to:

● clarify ideas
● identify the key concepts
● use synonyms and terms
● vary the search services
● vary the sources
● open/close the search
● aim for *enough*, not *all*
● evaluate sites.

Help in searching

Use Figure 10.1 below to itemise the concepts for which you are searching and some likely synonyms for each concept; the synonym may be as simple as specifying alternative spellings: *-ise* and *-ize* or *color* and *colour*, for example. Remember, the database will not know that you are not American and therefore spell words differently, and specifying one style of spelling may skew the source of the records retrieved.

Using Boolean searching

To get the most from Boolean searching it is important to understand what happens when each term is used to improve a search (Figs 10.2 and 10.3).

Concept	1:	2:	3:
Synonym 1	or:	or:	or:
Synonym 2	or:	or:	or:
Synonym 3	or:	or:	or:

Ordinarily, compose your query with brackets around synonyms with the OR, and use the AND to link the concepts:

(____ OR ____) AND (____ OR ____) AND (____ OR ____)

Figure 10.1 Itemising the search concepts (Courtesy of Mark Kerr, South Bank University).

Information technology and systems in communication

and	&
or	|
not	!
near	~

Figure 10.2 Boolean operands (Courtesy of Mark Kerr, South Bank University).

OR

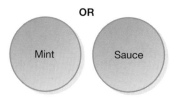

OR *broadens* a search, including all records containing at least one of the search terms. **OR** is good for linking related terms or synonyms to retrieve as much relevant material as possible.

AND

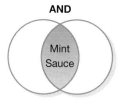

AND *narrows* a search, including only those records which contain both search terms. **AND** is good for refining a search to the specific topic being researched.

NOT

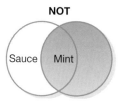

NOT (or **AND NOT**) also *narrows* a search, excluding records with specific terms. However, if the word excluded was only mentioned in passing in an otherwise useful record, it would still be excluded, so use this carefully.

Figure 10.3

Combining terms

Boolean logic uses algebra: terms are combined in the same way as mathematical terms. Place each term in brackets, then combine the bracketed terms to allow highly specific searches to be built up:

> ((lamb OR mutton OR sheep) AND (mint OR rosemary OR mustard)) AND NOT (restaurant OR menu)

Evaluation of material

Once we have found the required material we need to assess it. The basic steps for assessment are listed below.

- Who provided it and why?
- Is it accurate and up to date?
- Copyright issues
- Scope and coverage
- Are sources official?
- Is the information free?

These features are not in any particular order of importance and may change depending on the type of search you are performing.

CONCLUSION

The impact of ICT in recent years has been considerable and the successful use of them can significantly aid internal and external communications for an organisation. This is critical in communication between health professionals.

By applying simple protocols and processes, individuals and organisations can enhance the use of these technologies and consequently optimise the exchange of information and provide a good impression of their institution.

The effective use and integration of the telephone, fax and email can provide an infrastructure for co-working which can increase the efficiency of data exchange. Consequently, enabling necessary information to be available to clinicians will enhance the care provided for our patients.

The use of electronic communication in the provision of health care will only increase and it is the health care professional's duty not only to be aware of these developments but also to be efficient in their use and application.

References

NHS Information Authority 1998 NHSIA – Information for Health contents page. http://www.nhsia.nhs.uk/def/pages/info4health/contents.asp (accessed August 2001)

Sherwood K 2000 A beginner's guide to effective email. http://www.webfoot.com/advice/email.top.html (accessed August 2001)

Trigano AJ, Azoulay A, Rochdi M, Campillo A 1999 Electromagnetic interference of external pacemakers by walkie-talkies and digital cellular phones: experimental study. Pacing and Clinical Electrophysiology 22(4 Pt 1): 588–593

Further reading

Business Communications Review 2001 BCR Enterprises Inc. http://www.bcr.com/

Information technology and systems in communication

Electronic Privacy Information Centre 2001 http://www.epic.org/ (accessed August 2001)

Flynn T, Flynn N 2000 Writing effective email. Kogan Page, London

Harvard Business Review 1999 Harvard Business Review on effective communication. Harvard Business School Press, Boston, Massachusetts

NHS Information Authority 1998 NHSIA – Information for Health. http://www.nhsia.nhs.uk/def/pages/info4health/contents.asp (accessed August 2001)

Radiological Society of North America 2001 Integrated health care environment. http://www.rsna.org/IHE/index.shtml (accessed August 2001)

Sherwood K 2000 A beginner's guide to effective email. http://www.webfoot.com/advice/email.top.html (accessed August 2001)

Stallings W, Van Slyke R 2000 Business data communications, 3rd edn. http://williamstallings.com/BDC3e.html (accessed August 2001)

Stanton S 1996 Mastering communication. Palgrave, London

Tannen D 1996 Talking from nine to five. Virago, London

Tierney E 1997 30 minutes to boost your communication skills. Kogan Page, London

Resources

BioMedNet – http://www.bmn.com
Department of Health – http://www.open.gov.uk/health
Google – http://www.google.com
Health Service Journal – http://www.hsj.co.uk
UK Practice net – http://www.ukpractice.net

The elements of communication

Application **10:1**

Mike Tatlow

Data protection explained

The following information provides a detailed breakdown of the principles that underpin data protection legislation. While not everyone will require such detailed knowledge it is useful to know something of this important area as the archiving, transmission and use of electronic communication assume a more important role in our working lives.

SECTION A

SCHEDULE 1: THE DATA PROTECTION PRINCIPLES

1. Personal data shall be processed fairly and lawfully, and, in particular, shall not be processed unless-
   (a) at least one of the conditions in Schedule 2 is met, and
   (b) in the case of sensitive personal data at least one of the conditions in Schedule 3 is also met.
2. Personal data shall be obtained only for one or more specified and lawful purposes, and shall not be further processed in any manner incompatible with that purpose or those purposes.
3. Personal data shall be adequate, relevant and not excessive in relation to the purpose or purposes for which they are processed.
4. Personal data shall be accurate and, where necessary, kept up to date.
5. Personal data processed for any purpose or purposes shall not be kept for longer than is necessary for that purpose or those purposes.
6. Personal data shall be processed in accordance with the rights of data subjects under this Act.
7. Appropriate technical and organisational measures shall be taken against unauthorised or unlawful processing of personal data and

against accidental loss or destruction of, or damage to, personal data.

8. Personal data shall not be transferred to a country or territory outside the European Economic Area unless that country or territory ensures an adequate level of protection for the rights and freedoms of data subjects in relation to the processing of personal data.

Part II of Schedule 1 of the Act provides a more detailed interpretation of these provisions which should be consulted as appropriate.

SECTION B

SCHEDULE 2: CONDITIONS RELEVANT FOR THE PURPOSES OF THE FIRST PRINCIPLE: PROCESSING OF ANY PERSONAL DATA

1. The data subject has given his consent to the processing.
2. The processing is necessary-
   (a) for the performance of a contract to which the data subject is a party, or
   (b) for the taking of steps at the request of the data subject with a view to entering into a contract.
3. The processing is necessary for compliance with any legal obligation to which the data controller is subject, other than an obligation imposed by contract.
4. The processing is necessary to protect the vital interests of the data subject.
5. The processing is necessary-
   (a) for the administration of justice
   (b) for the exercise of any functions conferred on any person by or under any enactment
   (c) for the exercise of any functions of the Crown, a Minister of the Crown or a government department
   (d) for the exercise of any other functions of a public nature exercised in the public interest by any person.
6. (1) The processing is necessary for the purpose of legitimate interests pursued by the data controller or by the third party or parties to whom the data are disclosed, except where the processing is unwarranted in any particular case by reason of prejudice to the rights and freedoms or legitimate interests of the data subject.

(2) The secretary of state may by order specify particular circumstances in which this condition is, or is not, to be taken to be satisfied.

SECTION C

SCHEDULE 3: CONDITIONS RELEVANT FOR THE PURPOSES OF THE FIRST PRINCIPLE: PROCESSING OF SENSITIVE PERSONAL DATA

1. The data subject has given his explicit consent to the processing of the personal data.

2. (1) The processing is necessary for the purposes of exercising or performing any right or obligation which is conferred or imposed by law on the data controller in connection with employment.

(2) The secretary of state may by order-
(a) exclude the application of sub-paragraph (1) in such cases as may be specified, or
(b) provide that, in such cases as may be specified, the condition in sub-paragraph (1) is not to be regarded as satisfied unless such further conditions as may be specified in the order are also satisfied.

3. (1) The processing is necessary-
(a) in order to protect the vital interests of the data subject or another person, in a case where-
(i) consent cannot be given by or on behalf of the data subject, or,
(ii) the data controller cannot reasonably be expected to obtain the consent of the data subject, or
(b) in order to protect the vital interests of another person, in a case where consent by or on behalf of the data subject has been unreasonably withheld.

4. The processing-
(a) is carried out in the course of its legitimate activities by any body or association which-
(i) is not established or conducted for profit, and
(ii) exists for political, philosophical, religious or trade-union purposes,
(b) is carried out with appropriate safeguards for the rights and freedoms of data subjects,
(c) relates only to individuals who either are members of the body or association or have regular contact with it in connection with its purposes, and

(d) does not involve disclosure of the personal data to a third party without the consent of the data subject.

5. The information contained in the personal data has been made public as a result of steps deliberately taken by the data subject.

6. The processing-
- (a) is necessary for the purpose of, or in connection with, any legal proceedings (including prospective legal proceedings),
- (b) is necessary for the purpose of obtaining legal advice, or
- (c) is otherwise necessary for the purposes of establishing, exercising or defending legal rights.

7. (1) The processing is necessary-
- (a) for the administration of justice,
- (b) for the exercise of any functions conferred on any person by or under an enactment, or
- (c) for the exercise of any functions of the Crown, a Minister of the Crown or a government department.

(2) The secretary of state may by order-
- (a) exclude the application of sub-paragraph (1) in such cases as may be specified, or
- (b) provide that, in such cases as may be specified, the condition in sub-paragraph (1) is not to be regarded as satisfied unless such further conditions as may be specified in the order are also satisfied.

8. (1) The processing is necessary for medical purposes and is undertaken by-
- (a) a health professional, or
- (b) a person who in the circumstances owes a duty of confidentiality which is equivalent to that which would arise if that person were a health professional.

(2) In this paragraph "medical purposes" includes the purposes of preventative medicine, medical diagnosis, medical research, the provision of care and treatment and the management of health care services.

9. (1) The processing-
- (a) is of sensitive personal data consisting of information as to racial or ethnic origin,
- (b) is necessary for the purpose of identifying or keeping under review the existence or absence of equality of opportunity or treatment between persons of different racial or ethnic origins, with a view to enabling such equality to be promoted or maintained, and
- (c) is carried out with appropriate safeguards for the rights and freedoms of data subjects.

(2) The secretary of state may by order specify circumstances in which processing falling within sub-paragraph (1)(a) and (b) is, or is not, to be taken for the purposes of sub-paragraph (1)(c)

The elements of communication

to be carried out with the appropriate safeguards for the rights and freedoms of data subjects.

10. The personal data are processed in circumstances specified in an order made by the secretary of state for the purposes of this paragraph.

Application 10:2

Catriona King

Information technology and communication in practice

If communication is to be effective in any setting and in particular in the health care setting where confusion can easily occur because of the emotive issues involved, it is essential to take into account the needs of the individual or group with whom clinical professionals are trying to communicate.

This may entail taking into account differences in age, sex, culture, religion and ability. Communication should therefore take place in a manner and format that best suits those being communicated with so that the impact of the communication is not lost.

In the training of health care professionals every effort should be made to try to make clinicians aware that the person with whom they are communicating may have different needs and perspectives and, as far as possible, try to adapt to these. The following example of clinical practice illustrates how information technology combined with perceptions based on scarce experience of cultural issues prevent effective communication.

Case study 10.2.1

When I was at the end of my trainee GP year (now GP registrar year) in the late 1980s I was working in a very successful practice with two branches in central London. We had a high concentration of patients from Saudi Arabia who along with their children came to the practice for treatment and consultation.

One of the new doctors in the practice was a young man in his early thirties, Welsh and unmarried. He had not trained in London or any large city and was from a relatively religious background. He had also not carried out any postgraduate training in obstetrics or gynaecology. He had many strengths, one of which was his computer literacy which was a great asset to the practice.

His consulting room was immediately adjacent to the GP trainees' room and his patients shared a waiting room with my own.

On the occasion in question I had finished my surgery and was writing up notes in my room when I heard a commotion outside. When I looked outside I discovered a young woman crying and the new doctor and practice nurse trying to calm her down. I asked if I could help and the new doctor looked pleadingly and asked me if I could take the young woman into my room and talk to her. This I did.

She was, I discovered, 23 and she dressed in Western clothes but her facial appearance indicated she was of either Mediterranean or Arabic origin. Her name seemed to be Arabic in origin.

These facts alone, through my knowledge of the area and the recognised behaviour of these young women, alerted me to certain possible health habits and what are considered to be typical behaviours.

I asked her where her family originated from. She confirmed it was Saudi Arabia and that she had been born in London but lived with her large extended family. Further questioning indicated that she was a practising Muslim. Although she dressed in a Western manner I was alerted to differences that might apply to her outlook when compared to other 23-year-old London girls.

I talked to her at length using all the techniques of facilitation, active listening and, most importantly, eye contact that I had been taught. Eventually she stopped crying and told me what had happened.

She had made an appointment to see a female doctor but the receptionist that day had told her that she was seeing Dr X and to take a seat upstairs in the waiting room.

The young woman was called by the new male doctor. On arriving in his consulting room she was too shy to tell him that she felt uncomfortable about seeing him. He was unaware of her likely religious and cultural outlook due to his relative lack of experience. When he went into his consulting room he did the first thing he felt comfortable with: he turned to his computer. The young Saudi woman became even more shy and could not articulate what she had come for (which was in fact a problem with a skin rash).

He assumed on seeing her shyness that she had a gynaecological problem which was making her embarrassed and he became embarrassed himself. He asked her to undress behind the curtain and went to get a nurse chaperone. When he returned he consulted his computer and noted that she had never had a smear and decided to do one. He felt secure in the knowledge thus gained from the computer but found himself confronted with the woman crying (she had not undressed) and that is where I came in.

(*Cont.*)

In summary

I checked her rash (which was eczema) and explained why the mistake had occurred. I also explained to her about smears (however, as I thought from my knowledge of her religious and cultural background , she had never been sexually active despite her modern looks) and everything was cleared up quickly and she went away happy.

The male doctor spent some time following the incident learning about his local patient population, differences in culture and religion and how they influence health behaviours. He was also sent on a family planning course locally and was asked to stop hiding behind his computer screen!

The practice manager spoke to the receptionist about patient and customer management. It is to be hoped that future potentially inflammatory situations will be avoided.

This example of poor communication and overreliance on a computer might have escalated into a formal complaint against the doctor concerned. This can be referred to the General Medical Council (GMC) which is unfortunate when the situation has arisen through a misunderstanding. All health care professionals need to bear this in mind as the UKCC (NMC) and other professional bodies are taking an increasingly dim view of situations where patients face abuse or poor health care as a result of negligence or, in this case, lack of experience. Overreliance on technical equipment will not provide a defence as health care professionals need to see the patient as their prime source of information, with technology being used to support their judgement.

Index

Index